ANIMAL HOSPITAL

SCIENTISTS AT WORK

ANIMAL HOSPITAL

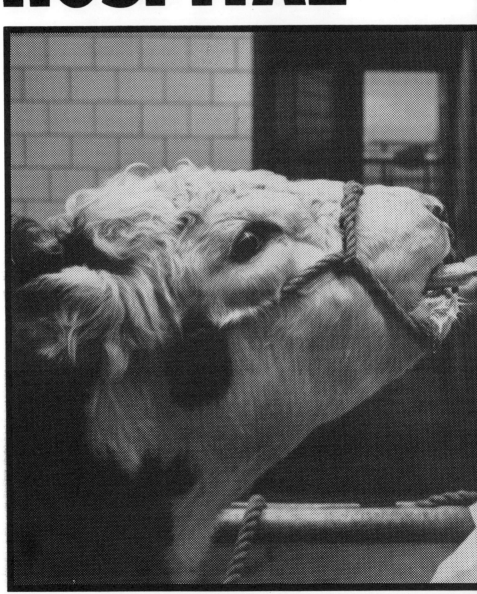

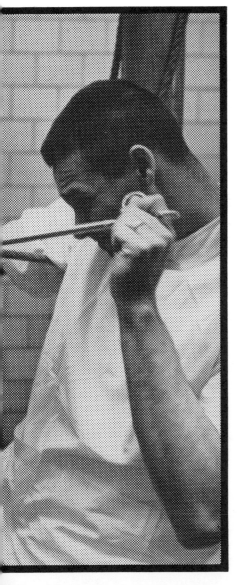

MELVIN BERGER

THE JOHN DAY COMPANY
NEW YORK

An Intext Publisher

OTHER TITLES IN THE SCIENTISTS AT WORK SERIES
South Pole Station
The National Weather Service
Oceanography Lab

Berger, Melvin.
    Animal hospital.
    (His Scientists at work)
    SUMMARY: *Discusses the varied activities of veterinarians and their assistants in animal hospitals and of researchers in animal medicine.*
    Bibliography: p.
    1. Veterinary hospitals—Juvenile literature. 2. Veterinary medicine—Juvenile literature. [1. Veterinary hospitals. 2. Veterinary medicine] I. Title.
SF604.5.B47   636.089   72-2418
ISBN: 0-381-99941-6 (reinforced edition)

Second Impression

The John Day Company, 257 Park Avenue South, New York, N.Y. 10010

Published on the same day in Canada by Longman Canada Limited.

Printed in the United States of America

For Bobby Scalcione

CONTENTS

ACKNOWLEDGMENTS

In doing research for this book I visited several animal hospitals and laboratories, as well as the New York State Veterinary College. I wish to thank the many veterinarians and researchers who spoke with me, for their kindness and help, for their interest in the writing of this book, and for their valued comments on the completed manuscript. I particularly want to express my gratitude to Drs. Robert B. Altman, William D. DeHoff, James A. Baker, N. Bruce Haynes, and Jules Markofsky.

FOREWORD

The purpose of the veterinary, or animal, hospital is exactly the same as that of the human hospital. They both exist to help the sick and the injured, and to keep those that are healthy in good health. In the veterinary hospital the doctors, called veterinarians, treat animal patients. In the human hospital the doctors treat human beings.

There is great drama and excitement in the veterinary hospital. The veterinarians must often stop what they are doing and rush to save the life of an animal badly injured in an accident. They apply all of their knowledge and their skills to help their patients.

The veterinarian gets deep feelings of satisfaction when he relieves the pain or cures the disease of his animal patients. How gratifying it is to be able to tell a worried pet owner that his loved pet is healthy again!

In recent years the pet population has been growing by leaps and bounds. The need for more veterinarians and for more veterinary hospitals is greater than ever.

Through this book you will get to know about animal hospitals. The interesting photographs and the clear text show you the inside workings of an animal hospital. The book also describes the many activities of the veterinarians at work. It shows the new medical equipment and the modern techniques that they use to give your pet—whether dog, cat, bird, chimpanzee, snake, or mouse—the very best medical care that is possible today.

ROBERT B. ALTMAN, D.V.M.
Merrick, New York

ANIMAL HOSPITAL

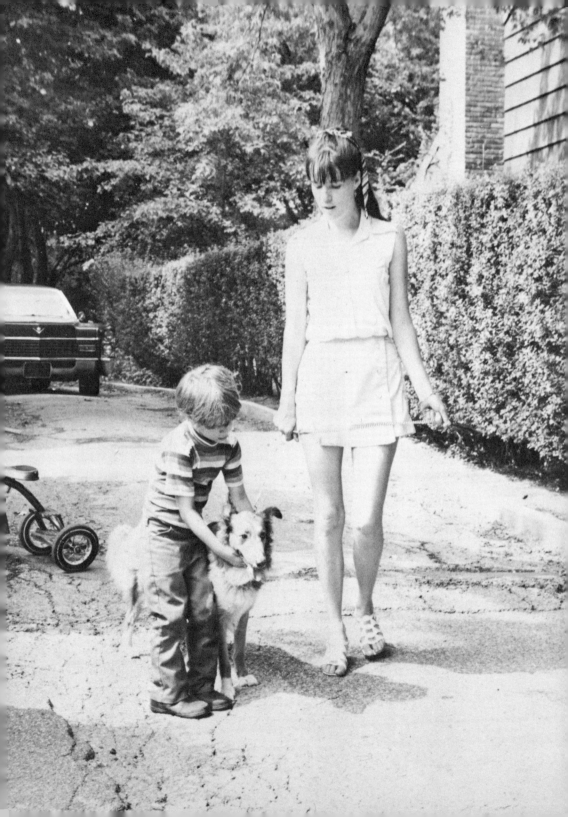

THE ANIMAL HOSPITAL

Princess lay quietly in the driveway. She did not bark. She did not jump up when Bobby came out to play with her. The only part of her that moved were her sad eyes.

Bobby became frightened. He ran into the house to call his mother. She rushed out with Bobby. In a glance she saw that the dog was sick. She told Bobby that they had better take Princess to the animal hospital.

At the animal hospital there are doctors who treat sick dogs, cats, and other pet animals. Although there are also animal hospitals that treat large animals, such as horses and cows, most ani-

Bobby became frightened when Princess
did not jump up and play with him.

mal hospitals care for the small animals that people keep as pets.

The doctors who work in animal hospitals are called veterinarians. Sometimes they are called vets for short. Just as medical doctors treat people, veterinarians treat animals.

In a few minutes, Bobby, his mother, and Princess were in the car and on their way to the animal hospital.

The hospital is a large, white building. When they arrived, they went right into the waiting room. Bobby sat down on a chair, and Princess stretched out at his feet. His mother went over to the lady

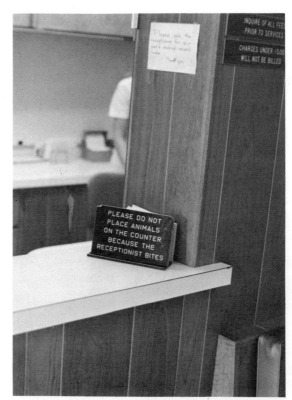

The funny sign is near the receptionist's desk in the animal hospital.

Melvin Berger

16

who was sitting at a desk in the corner of the waiting room. She is the receptionist. It is her job to greet the people who come into the hospital and to make appointments for the veterinarians to see the sick animals.

Bobby's mother gave her name to the receptionist and asked to have one of the veterinarians examine the dog. The receptionist wrote down the name and asked her to sit down and wait until a veterinarian was free to help her.

The animal hospital is a busy place. There are several veterinar-

Very sick animals must stay in the hospital.
They are kept in stainless steel cages.

Melvin Berger

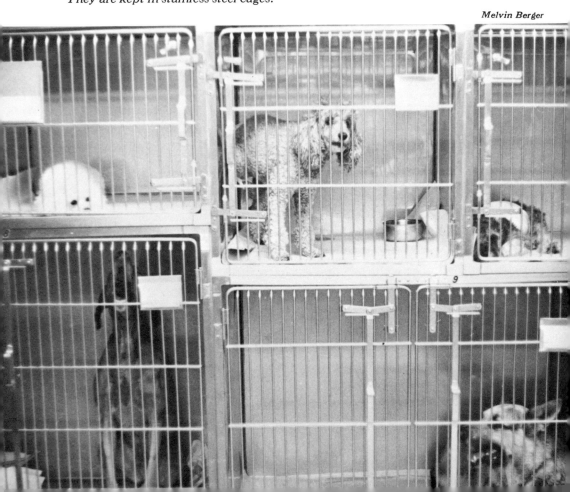

ians and their helpers at work. In one room, a veterinarian is examining a dog's ear to see if there is an infection. In another room, a veterinarian is changing the bandage on a bad wound that a cat got in a fight with another cat. In the operating room of the hospital, still another veterinarian is operating on a dog's leg. He is joining together the bones that were broken when the dog was hit by a car. In the X-ray room, a veterinarian is taking X-ray pictures of a sick parakeet. And in the laboratory of the animal hospital, a veterinarian is doing tests on blood taken from a rabbit, trying to find the exact cause of its illness.

Several rooms in the animal hospital are lined with stainless steel cages. These are the wards of the hospital. Each cage has an animal inside. The animals who are here are very sick. They must stay in the hospital until they are well again.

In a little while, a veterinarian came through a door and into the waiting room. He was wearing a long, white coat. He nodded to Bobby and his mother. But he was mostly interested in the dog.

"What is her name?" he asked.

"Princess," Bobby said softly.

The veterinarian bent down. "Hi, Princess," he said to the dog. He petted her on the head. He scratched her behind the ears. He smoothed down the fur on her back. Princess had seemed frightened when the doctor first came over. But now she relaxed.

Then, very gently, the veterinarian took the leash that Bobby had been holding. Moving slowly and talking quietly to Princess at the same time, he led the dog back through the door. Bobby and his mother followed.

They entered a small, brightly-lit room. In the center of the

*The monkey is afraid
to let go of his owner.*

Melvin Berger

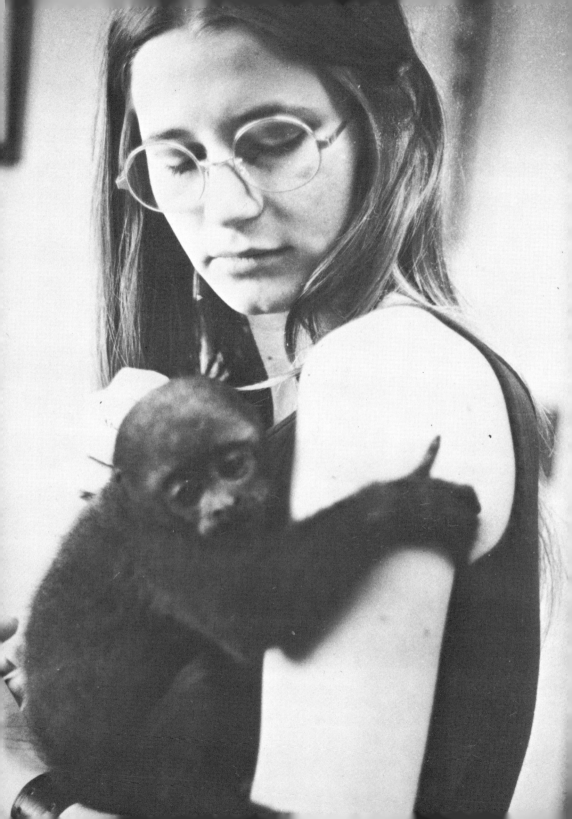

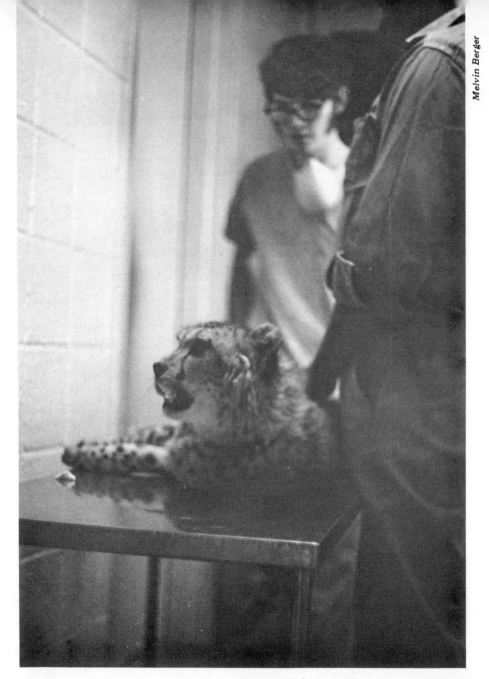

*The veterinarian never knows what animals will
show up at the animal hospital.
Here is a sick cheetah he had to treat.*

room was a shiny metal table. The veterinarian picked Princess up and placed her on the table. She did not bark or struggle.

Without startling her, the veterinarian began to examine Princess. He looked into her ears and mouth. He felt at various spots around her body. All the while, he asked Bobby's mother questions about the pet's health and behavior.

Finally, the doctor finished the examination. He explained that some germs in the dog's stomach were making her sick. But he said that it was not serious at all.

He gave Bobby's mother a bottle of medicine for Princess. "Give her a spoonful every morning. In two or three days, Princess will be as good as new," he said, as he led them back to the waiting room.

Bobby made it his job to give Princess her medicine. Every

The animal hospital gets some strange requests.
One boy's pet mouse "dide," and
he asked the veterinarian to take care of the body.

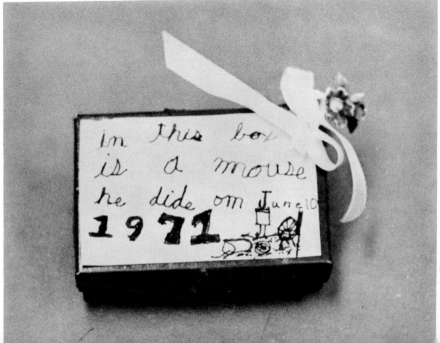

Melvin Berger

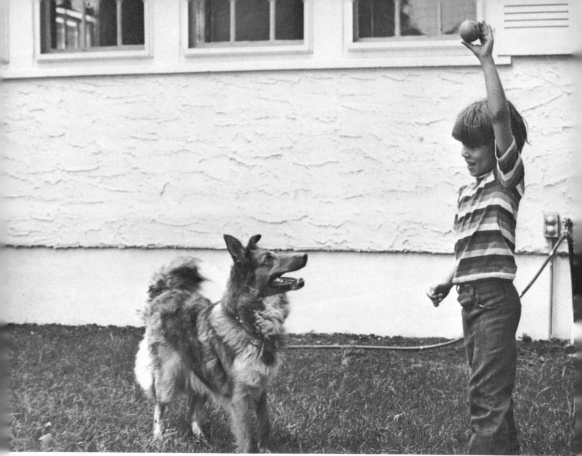

Melvin Berger

The veterinarian cured Princess.
Now she enjoys playing ball with Bobby.

morning he gave her a spoonful of the liquid medicine that the veterinarian had given them.

By the third day, Princess was her usual, frisky self. She jumped up and barked when Bobby came out to play with her. When he threw a ball, she scampered after it and brought it back for more.

Not only had the veterinarian cured Princess. He had also made Bobby a very happy boy.

THE ANIMAL DOCTOR

Are you one of the 50 million people in the United States that owns a cat or dog? Are you among the 20 million people who own a pet bird? Do you have a pet rabbit, gerbil, monkey, hamster, lizard, snake, or any other animal? If you do, then the chances are good that you have visited an animal hospital and that you have met an animal doctor—a veterinarian.

A veterinarian is a highly trained doctor who deals with the diseases of animals. It is his or her job to "diagnose, treat, operate, or prescribe for any animal disease, pain, injury, deformity, or physical condition." "Animal" includes all living creatures except humans.

There are nearly 30,000 veterinarians at work in this country. Almost every one of them started to become a veterinarian very early in life. As a child he loved animals. His family usually had a pet of some sort. Perhaps he had a pet of his own that he fed and cared for. Many veterinarians grew up on farms, where they helped out with the farm animals. Most of them had the experience of nursing a sick or injured animal back to health.

The young person who grew up to be a veterinarian was probably always interested in animals. If he found a stray wild animal or bird, he took care of it; he fed it and tried to find its home. He tried to learn as much as he could about animals of all kinds.

As a teenager, the veterinarian-to-be may have worked with animals after school or during the summers. He may have helped out at an animal hospital or at a kennel. Perhaps he handled the animals on a farm or ranch. Maybe he did chores in a zoo or a pet shop. Almost every veterinarian showed an early interest in animals and spent some time working with animals when he was young.

The person who wants to be a veterinarian usually majors in science in high school and college. He takes many courses in biology, chemistry, and physics. After three years of college, the student applies to go to one of the eighteen veterinary colleges in the United States.

It is quite difficult to be accepted in one of these schools. In some colleges, about ten students apply for each one that can be accepted. The student is selected on the basis of his college marks, the strength of his desire to become a veterinarian, and signs of an early interest in animals.

During the four years in veterinary school, the student spends

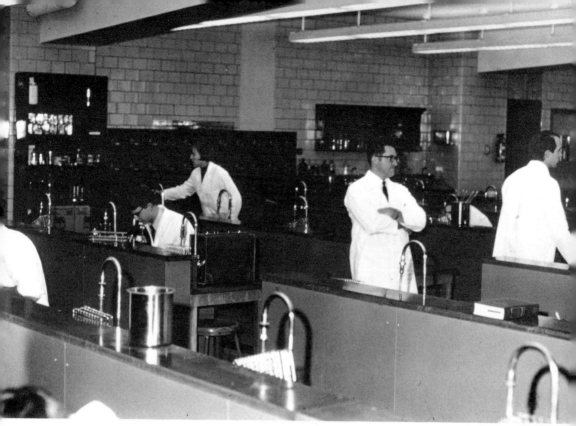

*The veterinary student spends many hours learning chemistry
and biology in the college laboratories.*

about 5,000 hours in classes. In the first years the courses cover the basic sciences, particularly the anatomy, chemistry, nutrition, and growth of different types of animals. The student takes courses that cover every aspect of the diseases of animals. He learns what causes different diseases and how to prevent the spread of disease. He is taught to recognize diseases in sick animals and to know what drugs or treatments to use in curing them. He finds out how to pre-

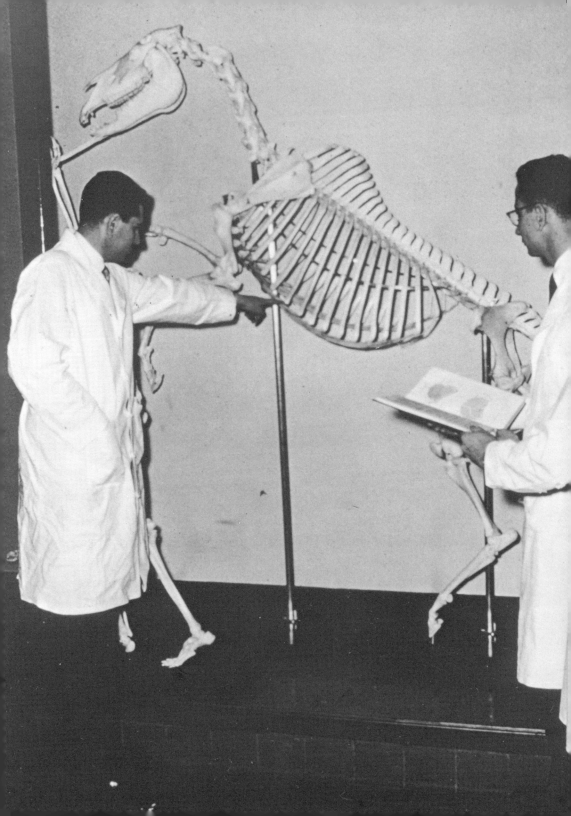

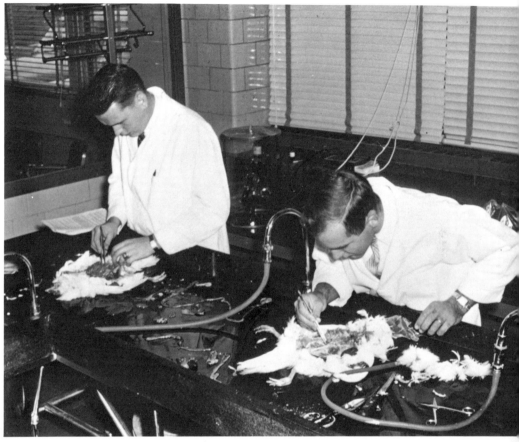

These veterinary students are doing autopsies on dead chickens to find the cause of death.

The skeleton of a horse is used to teach anatomy in the veterinary college.

Melvin Berger

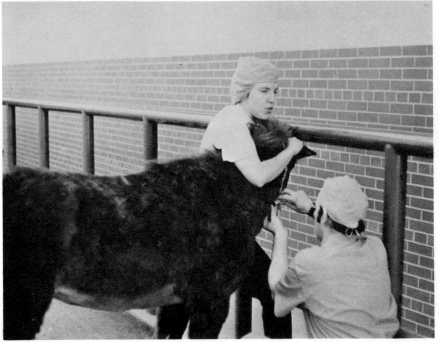

*It takes two student veterinarians to hold
the pony as he is given a sedative to calm him before surgery.
Notice that his belly has been shaved.*

pare drugs and to take X-ray pictures. He spends many hours in
the college laboratories studying the germs that cause disease and
the effect that they have on the animal's tissues and organs.

Later courses give the student a chance to work with sick animals. In the advanced classes he performs surgery and gives sick
animals the medicines or treatment that they need. The student
is taught how to apply his knowledge to all animals—from tiny pet

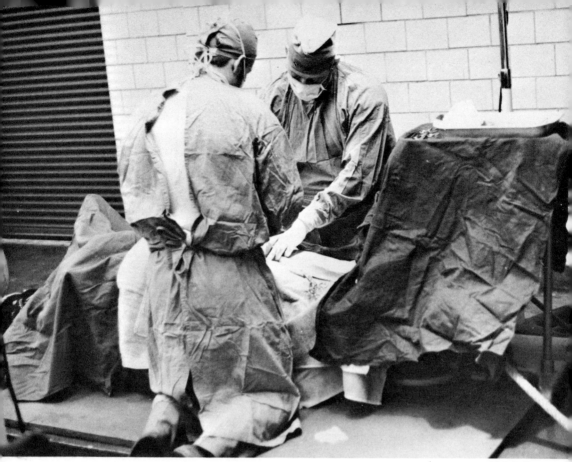

Two students work together in operating on the pony.

mice and hamsters, through dogs, cats, and birds, to cows, horses, and other large farm animals.

The veterinary student usually spends his final year at work in the animal hospital that is part of the veterinary college. Closely watched by his teachers, the student treats the sick animals that are brought to the hospital. The students are "on call" twenty-four hours a day. They must be ready to handle emergencies at any

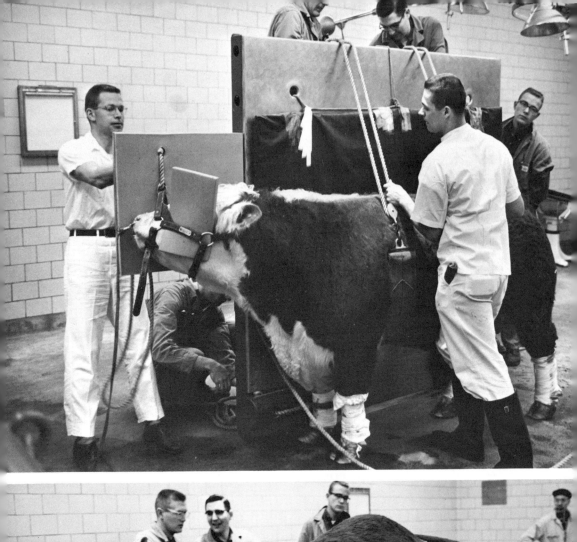
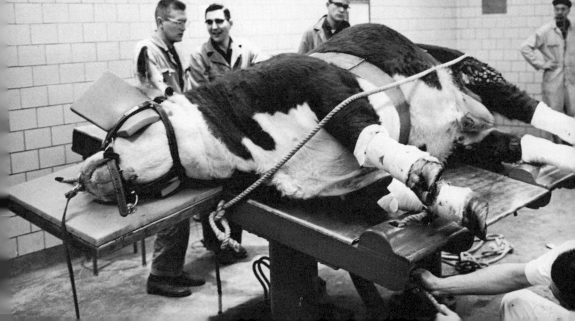

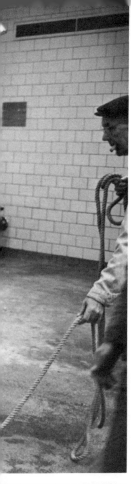

The students in surgery
at the veterinary college use
a tilting table for
operating on large animals.

Cornell University

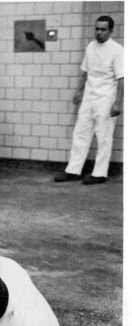

When the table is flat,
the students can begin to prepare
the animal for surgery.

Cornell University

31

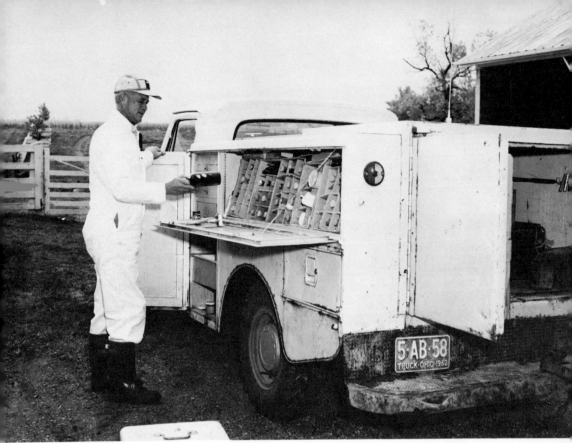

*This veterinarian uses a truck to carry
medicines and supplies when he visits sick farm animals.
Here he is getting a vaccine ready for a calf.*

time of the day or night. Most students attend class only one hour a day during the final year.

Veterinary students work very hard. They are serious and devoted to their goals. Very few fail or drop out. But many do have other interests besides animal medicine. Most veterinary colleges have clubs that are set up by the students for fun and relaxation.

Some students at the New York State Veterinary College, in Ithaca, New York, for example, play in small musical groups which rehearse once a week.

These hard-working students at veterinary schools also enjoy their little jokes. At the same college there is a tradition of playing a birthday prank each year on one of the favorite teachers, Dr. Francis Fox. One year the students released a flock of twenty chickens in his office. Another time they removed all the furniture, covered the floor with straw, and locked a calf in his room.

At the end of the four years in veterinary college, the student is awarded his degree—Doctor of Veterinary Medicine (D.V.M.). He has earned the right to be called doctor.

But he still cannot practice veterinary medicine. He must first pass a test given by the board of veterinary examiners of the state in which he wants to practice. The test covers all the knowledge and skills he will need to be a veterinarian. It takes in basic science and medical science. It also tests his ability to handle and to treat all types of sick animals. When he has passed this final hurdle, the veterinarian is ready at last to start his career.

He has a choice of several different fields of veterinary medicine. About 90 percent of the graduate veterinarians go into private practice. They usually work, at first, in the hospital of an older, more experienced veterinarian. Later on, they may open their own hospitals.

Some doctors go to work in animal hospitals that have a mixed practice. These hospitals treat both large and small animals. In one day, a veterinarian at work here may examine a herd of sick cows on a farm, clip the nails of a poodle in the office, and prescribe medicine for a canary that is losing its feathers.

ON THE FOLLOWING PAGES:
The cow does not seem to be enjoying this treatment by the veterinarian.

Cornell University

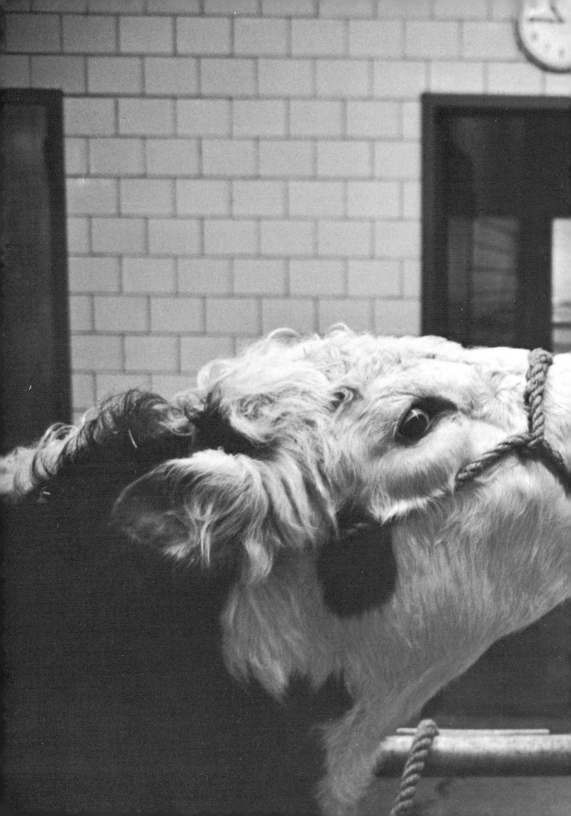

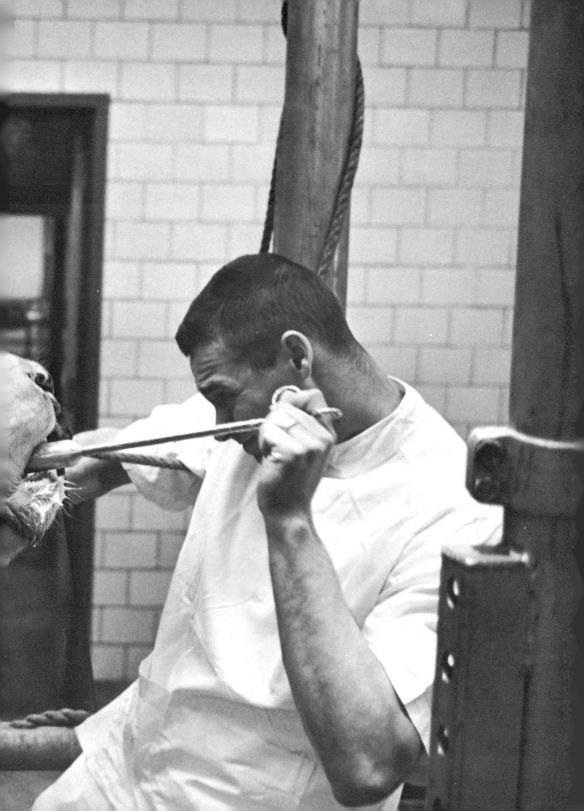

A good number of veterinarians find that they prefer treating small animals—dogs and cats and other household pets. They work in the small-animal hospitals that treat only these kinds of animals.

Working as a veterinarian in an animal hospital is a difficult, full-time job. The veterinarian spends several hours a day examining and treating the sick animals that owners bring to the hospital. He spends a few hours a day with the animals that are kept in the hospital. He checks their condition and gives them the medicines and treatment they need. Some days he spends an entire morning or afternoon doing surgery in the operating room.

At other times, the veterinarian has dozens of jobs to keep him busy. He takes an X-ray picture of a cat to see if her broken leg is healing correctly. In the laboratory he tests the blood of a sick cat to see exactly what type of germ is making him sick. He advises a worried owner on what foods to feed his overweight dog. He writes up reports and records on all the animals he has seen and treated. He studies the professional magazines and the new books that tell about the advances in veterinary science. And so on.

Also, the veterinarian must be ready at any time of the day or night to handle an emergency. As soon as the urgent call comes in, the veterinarian stops what he is doing—no matter if he is working at the hospital or relaxing at home—and rushes in to do what he can.

Most of the emergency calls are to treat animals that have been hit by cars. In the past, about half the animals the veterinarian cared for had been injured by autos. The percentage is much lower now. People have learned to use the leash more. But a few victims of auto accidents are still brought to a busy animal hospital every day. And these cases come in at all hours of the day and night.

As soon as the victim is brought in, the veterinarian swings into action. If there is serious bleeding, he works to stop the flow of blood. He cleans out and bandages any cuts and wounds. He gives drugs to avoid infection and to calm the animal who might be in a state of shock. He checks for broken bones and internal injuries that will require further treatment. Many badly hurt animals are saved because veterinarians are willing to rush to the hospital at a moment's notice to help them.

A veterinarian in an animal hospital works hard but he gets great rewards. He enjoys his work. He knows that he can relieve an animal of pain and suffering and at the same time bring happiness and comfort to its owner. Most veterinarians at work in animal hospitals would not trade places with anyone.

*Veterinarians are in charge of meat inspection
for the U.S. Department of Agriculture.*

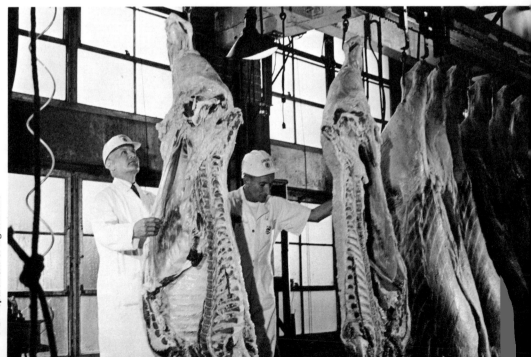

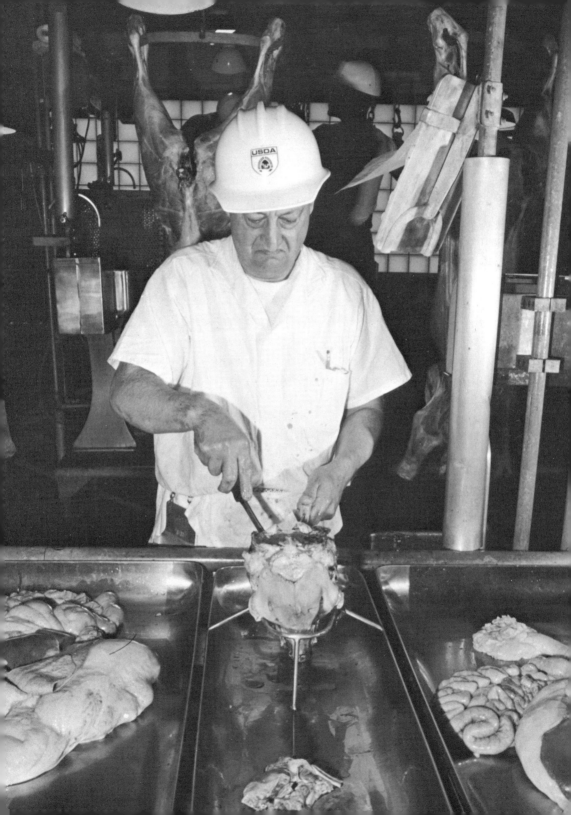

Some veterinarians, however, choose other fields of veterinary medicine. Many work for various government agencies. They watch over the animals that produce the food we eat. They visit farms and ranches to make sure that the cattle, hogs, and sheep, the chickens, turkeys, and ducks are free of disease and are being raised under healthy, wholesome conditions. They also make sure that the food products—the meat, poultry, eggs, and milk—are prepared and sold under the highest standards of cleanliness.

The veterinarian on the right draws a sample of blood
from a pig to check for disease.

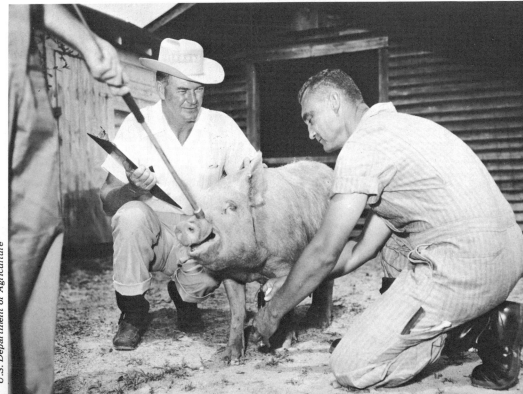

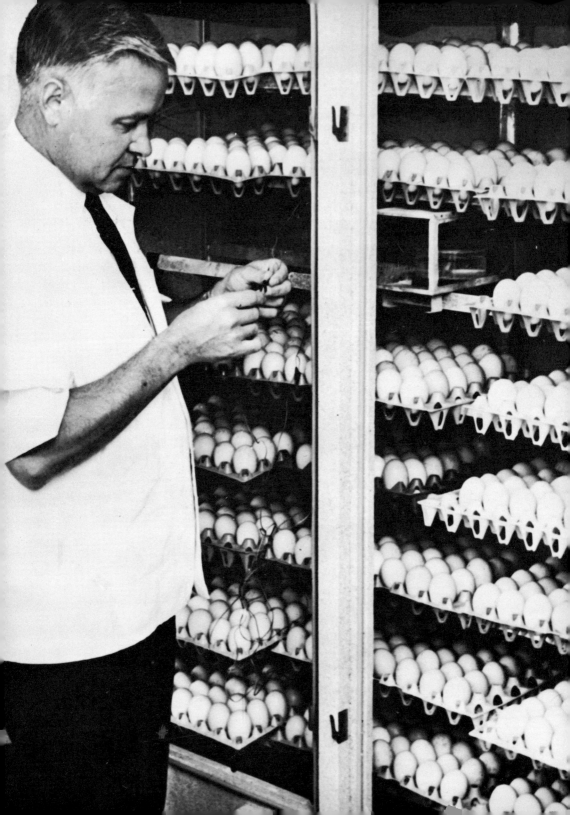

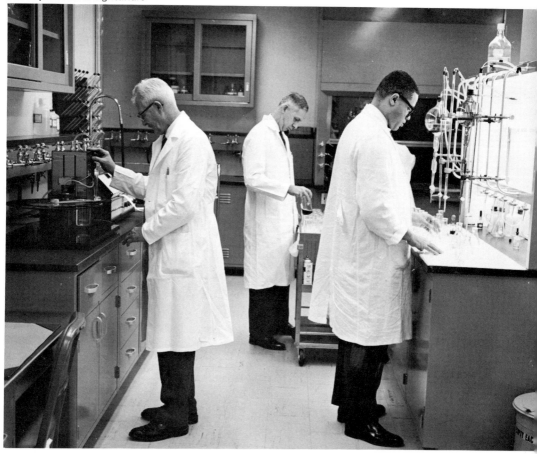

Research scientists study
meat products in a U.S. Department
of Agriculture laboratory.

This research veterinarian
is running an experiment
on the disease-causing germs
that infect eggs.

The biggest employer of veterinarians is the Department of Agriculture of the United States government. These veterinarians inspect all the meat, poultry, and animal products that are sold in this country. They also do research on farm animals, trying to eliminate disease and searching for improved methods of raising animals.

A certain number of veterinarians find work in medical research laboratories. In these laboratories they take care of the animals that are used in experiments to learn more about human and animal diseases, as well as to test new drugs. Other veterinarians work for zoos and on wildlife preserves. Some become teachers at veterinary colleges. A few veterinarians serve at racetracks, checking the condition of the horses before each race.

Doctors of veterinary medicine are in great demand today. More people now own house pets and horses than ever before. Veterinarians are needed to care for the health of these animals. The demand for meat and poultry continues to grow. Veterinarians are needed to look after the animals on farms and ranches. Consumers want to be sure that the meat and poultry they eat is wholesome and free of disease. Therefore, veterinarians are needed in government service, as well.

Each year, about 1,100 men and 100 women graduate as doctors of veterinary medicine. They join the veterinarians already in the field. Their work in expanding and improving the level of animal health care is for the benefit of all of us.

THE EXAMINATION ROOM

The small sign on the door of the animal hospital reads: OFFICE HOURS: 9-11 A.M., 2-4 P.M., AND BY APPOINTMENT.

The veterinarian spends many hours each day examining animal patients in the examination rooms of the hospital. The rooms that he uses are nearly bare. Each one usually has no more than a stainless steel table, a counter with a sink, and a glass-doored cabinet. The cabinet holds many bottles and boxes of medicines. It stores the supplies and instruments that the veterinarian uses in his examinations.

The veterinarian never knows what animal will be brought through the door of the examination room. And he has no idea what disease—if any—the animal will be suffering from. But the experienced veterinarians find that many examinations follow a similar course:

The animal that is brought to the veterinarian looks weak and tired. The owner tells the doctor that the pet suddenly started to vomit and is having severe diarrhea (frequent and loose bowel movements). But weakness, vomiting, and diarrhea are the symptoms of many different diseases. The veterinarian's first job, then, is to discover exactly which disease is causing the symptoms in this animal. He begins his examination.

The veterinarian has been studying the pet's appearance. Does he walk easily, or is he stiff in one or more legs? Does he show signs of pain as he walks? Does he shy away from the bright lights in the examination room? Does he show a normal interest in the new room and the new people that he is seeing?

As he thinks about these questions, the veterinarian dismisses many possible diseases at once. He narrows down the choices, as he tries to find the disease most likely to be causing the symptoms that he sees.

The veterinarian lifts the animal onto the table, so that he can examine him more closely. He looks carefully at the pet's face. Is there any discharge from his nose or ears? Are his eyes red or watery? Are his tongue and gums normal in color and appearance? Is he breathing too fast? Perhaps the veterinarian uses one of the instruments in the cabinet to help him look farther into the animal's ears or mouth.

The veterinarian pokes and pushes at various spots around the pet's body. He is on the lookout for any lumps or swelling. He also

The kitten is paying her first visit to the animal hospital. Here the veterinarian is checking her weight.

Cornell University

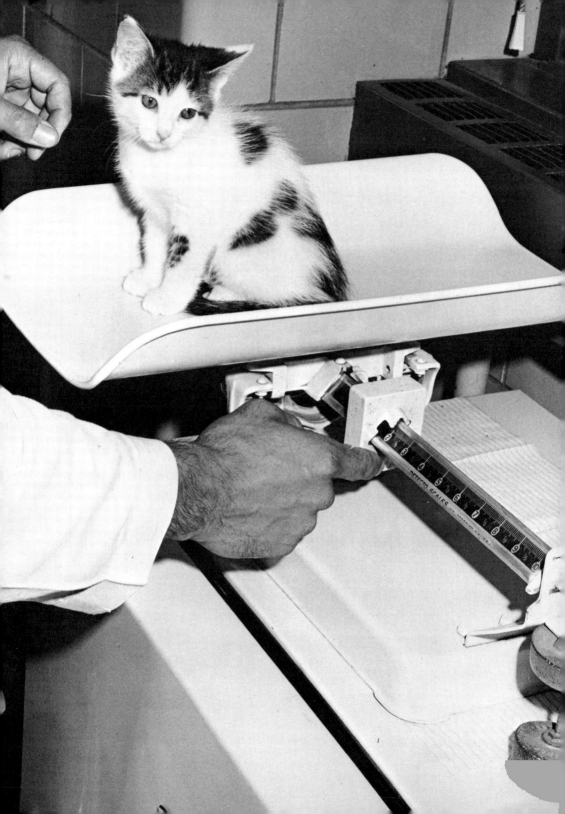

watches to see if the animal shows any signs of pain when he presses down in certain places.

The doctor passes his hand over the animal's fur. Is it shiny or dull? Are there any special problems? Is the animal shedding? Are there any bald spots? Are there any sores or wounds?

He uses a rectal thermometer to measure the pet's temperature. He uses a stethoscope to listen to the animal's heart and to other sounds inside the body.

During the examination the veterinarian also asks the owner many questions. He wants to know when the dog first became sick and what symptoms he showed. He finds out the age of the animal, its weight, and breeding. He asks about its general health and previous sicknesses, its behavior and its eating habits.

In his mind the veterinarian brings together the results of his examination and the information of the owner. He knows of thousands of animal diseases, their causes and symptoms. Now he wants to know exactly what is wrong with this animal. What is making this pet sick?

Could the sickness be caused by harmful bacteria?

Bacteria are invisible, one-celled plants that are found everywhere. They enter the animal's body every time he takes a breath, licks his fur, or gets a cut or scratch on his skin.

Most bacteria living in the bodies of animals and men and women do not cause disease. But there are a few types of bacteria that are dangerous and harmful. If these bacteria get inside the body, they attack the living tissue. Some bacteria multiply so rapidly in the tissue that it dies. Others produce poisons which also kill the tissue.

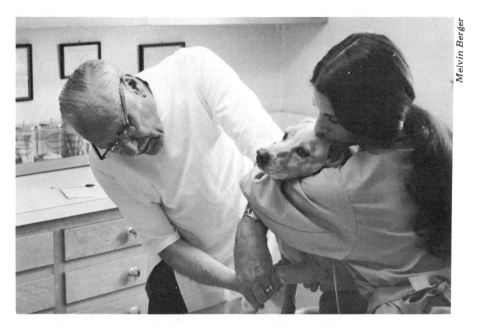

The veterinarian cannot ask the animal where it hurts.
He must find out by himself in the examination room.

The infections that follow injuries are usually the result of harmful bacteria. Fevers, food poisoning, and many diseases connected with breathing or eating and digesting food are caused by bacteria.

Could it be a virus-caused disease?

Viruses are even smaller than bacteria. Bacteria can be seen with an ordinary laboratory microscope. Viruses can be seen only by means of the powerful electron microscope.

Viruses attack the living cells in the animal's body. Part of the

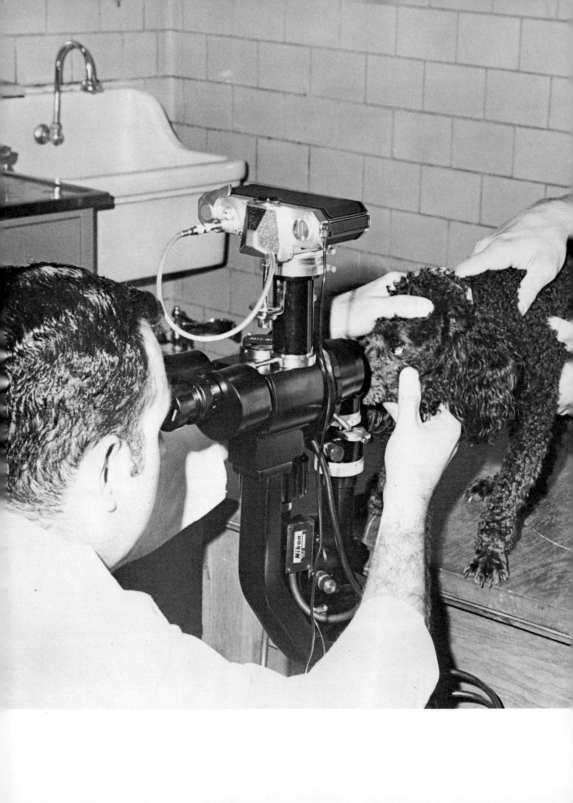

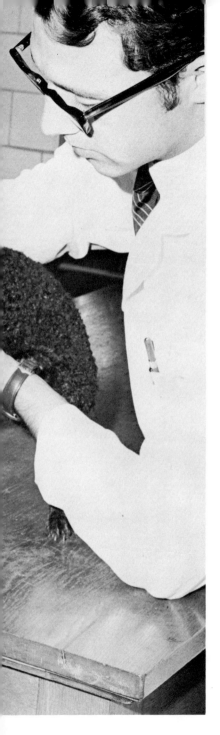

*The veterinarian uses
a complicated instrument,
called an ophthalmoscope, to
examine this dog's eyes.*

Cornell University

virus forces its way inside and takes over the working of the cell. In a few minutes the cell bursts apart. Hundreds of new viruses pour out of the destroyed cell. The new viruses then attack other cells, spreading the disease through the animal's body.

Some veterinarians believe that there are viruses that cause cells to multiply rapidly without stop. These cells form lumps in the animal's body, called cancers. Cancers can start growing almost anywhere and can quickly spread throughout the body. If the cancer does not stop growing by itself, or if it is not cut out by the veterinarian, it can lead to the death of the animal.

If the animal has a skin disease, the veterinarian wonders if the disease might be caused by a parasite.

Parasites are small animals or plants that live on larger animals. Several parasites may be found in the skin and fur of pet animals. The most common ones are the flea, the louse, the mite, and the tick.

The parasites vary in size from the mites, which can be seen only through a microscope, to the tick, which can be one-half inch long. But as small as they are, the parasites can cause the animal great pain and serious sickness.

Almost all of the parasites make the skin itch. The animal scratches. Scratching leads to cuts, bleeding, and sometimes infections. There is often a loss of hair and scaly red sores where the parasites are attached. And sometimes the parasite is carrying harmful bacteria or viruses. These can cause more serious illnesses.

Is the disease caused by worms?

Worms are parasites that live inside the animal's body. The ones that the veterinarian sees most often are the roundworm, the hookworm, the whipworm, and the tapeworm.

The worms give off poisons and destroy tissue and organs. If an animal has just a few worms, he may be weak and not have much appetite. If he has a large number of worms, the animal can be seriously sick.

Is there some other type of microscopic animal or plant that is causing the animal to be sick?

Is it a disease he inherited?

Is he sick because of a poor diet?

Is one part or organ of his body not doing its job?

The veterinarian combines science and art in making a diagnosis. The science is his vast knowledge of all animal diseases, their causes and symptoms. The art is in noticing little things about the sick animals and having right hunches about what makes animals sick.

By the time the examination is over, the veterinarian usually has a very good idea of what is wrong. Sometimes, however, the examination does not give him enough clues to allow him to name the exact disease and its cause.

He may need help from other parts of the animal hospital. He may ask for X-ray pictures that will show him the bones and organs inside the body. He may ask for laboratory tests that will give him information on the animal's condition that he could not get during the examination.

With this added information, the veterinarian is able to make a final diagnosis. But diagnosis of disease is only part of his work in the animal hospital. He also treats and cures the diseases that he finds. Very often, this is done in another part of the hospital— the treatment room.

THE TREATMENT ROOM

The treatment room looks very much like the examination room, except that it has more drugs and equipment for the doctor to use.

Most animal hospitals have several treatment rooms. Some are separate rooms. Here the veterinarian treats the animals that are brought in and taken home after treatment. Other treatment rooms are part of the wards. Here the veterinarian treats the animals who are so ill that they must stay in the hospital until they get better.

The veterinarian treats and cures the diseases of sick animals in the treatment room. But he also does the important work of preventing disease in healthy animals here.

For the first two months of a puppy's life, while he is nursing, the puppy is protected against a number of diseases by substances in the mother's milk. After that, the protection begins to disappear. Within a few weeks, the protection is gone. The puppy may become sick with one of the diseases that affect puppies.

Most veterinarians suggest that puppies be brought in for their first shot or injection when they are about two months old. Then they should have booster shots once a year. The shots guard the dog against three serious diseases—distemper, hepatitis and leptospirosis.

Distemper is caused by a virus infection. The first symptoms are a lack of appetite and periods of high fever. As the disease gets worse there is a discharge from the eyes and nose, severe diarrhea, and a hacking cough. Later there may be convulsions.

There is no drug to fight viruses. Therefore, there is no treatment for distemper. But the veterinarian can give the dog an injection that will prevent distemper. The shot is called a vaccine. There are a few kinds of distemper vaccine. They are made from either dead or very weak distemper viruses. When the vaccine is injected into the dog, it does not cause distemper. But it does lead his body to build up defenses against viruses of that type. Then, if some live distemper viruses invade his body, he is able to resist them.

The vaccine injection protects the dog for about a year. Then the protection begins to fade. That is why the veterinarian suggests that the dog be given a booster shot of vaccine once a year. That keeps the level of protection high at all times.

In the past, distemper was the most common disease and the biggest killer of dogs. Today, because veterinarians vaccinate so

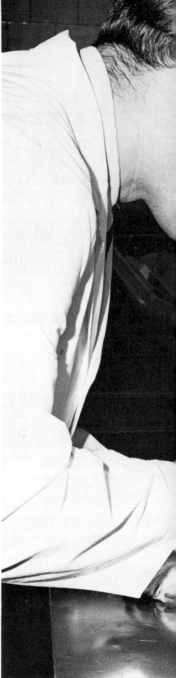

Cornell University

Melvin Berger

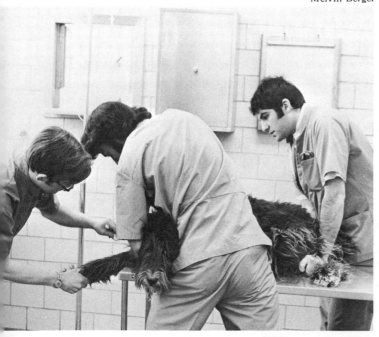

*It sometimes takes
three veterinarians to
hold a dog still
for its shots.*

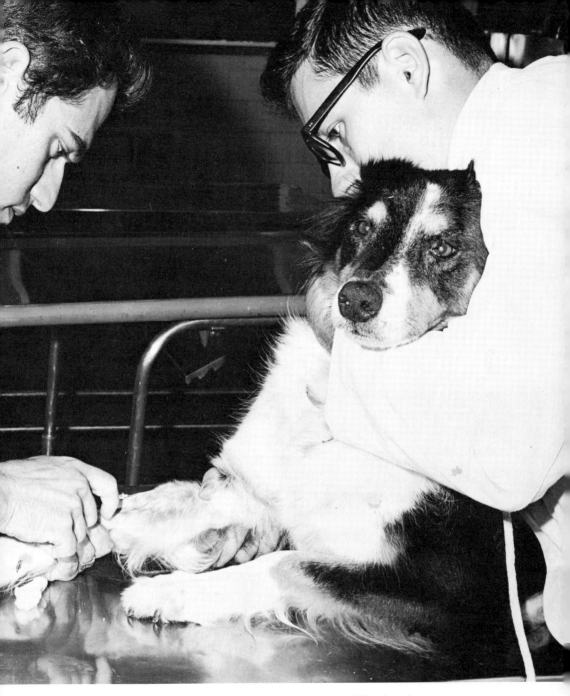

*The dog does not seem
to notice that he
is getting an injection
in his leg.*

many dogs, distemper is under better control. Still, it is very important that all dogs be vaccinated early. Dogs that are bought from other people should be vaccinated at once by the new owner's veterinarian. Many people buy dogs and are told they have been vaccinated. They should not rely on this and should have their own doctor give the dog injections.

Hepatitis is also a virus infection. It attacks the dog's liver and is very serious when it strikes dogs that are either very old or very young.

The early symptoms of hepatitis are similar to those of distemper. Later symptoms sometimes include vomiting, swollen tonsils, and pain when anyone or anything touches the dog's abdomen.

Hepatitis can be prevented by a vaccine that is prepared from viruses of the type that cause the disease. Usually the hepatitis vaccine is given at the same time as the distemper vaccine. It also requires a yearly booster shot to keep up the body's defenses.

Leptospirosis is a very contagious disease that is caused by bacteria. It is spread by the urine of either infected dogs or rats. Within a week or two, the sick animal shows symptoms similar to that of distemper or hepatitis. He has loss of appetite, weakness, high temperature, and vomiting. A few days later the temperature drops suddenly, the animal has difficulty breathing, and there is often a stiffness in the hind legs.

Some drugs can control the bacteria that cause leptospirosis if they are given early enough in the course of the disease. But the best way to fight leptospirosis is by a vaccine shot, once a year.

Usually the vaccines for distemper, hepatitis, and leptospirosis are given in one injection. Similar vaccines are also given to protect cats against some of the diseases they may catch.

The other common shot given by veterinarians protects the animal against rabies. Rabies is a virus disease that can attack man, as well as most animals. It is spread by the bite of an infected animal.

A dog with rabies is often called a mad dog. He growls and barks almost all the time and will sometimes attack without reason. In time, paralysis sets in, and the dog dies.

In city areas there is not too much danger of rabies. But in the countryside the danger of rabies is much greater. Almost all wild animals, including the fox and the skunk, can be infected with the

In the treatment area of a ward, some medicine is applied to a skin infection on a duck.

Melvin Berger

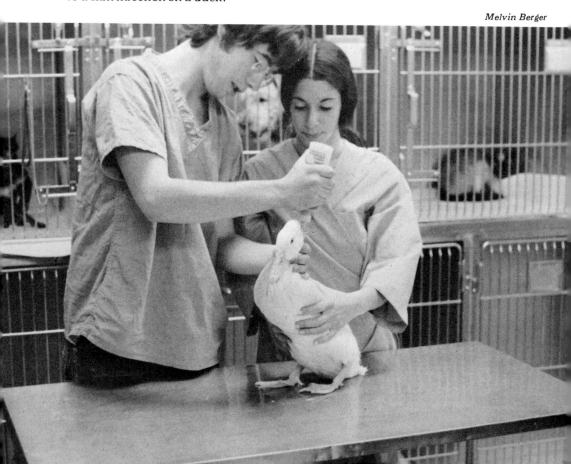

rabies virus. If the dog is bitten by one of these animals, he gets the disease and can then give it to any person he might bite. Veterinarians suggest that all dogs be given a rabies vaccine shot, usually at about six months of age. Booster shots should then be given every two or three years.

The diseases that the veterinarian cannot prevent he must try to cure. His strongest weapons in the fight against the diseases caused by bacteria are the modern miracle drugs, such as the antibiotics and sulfa drugs.

Penicillin is the most frequently used drug in today's animal hospital. Penicillin is a product that is given off by a type of mold. It is able to stop the growth of several different types of bacteria. Therefore it is an effective treatment for the many diseases caused by these bacteria.

Some of the drugs that the veterinarian prescribes are in pill or liquid form. He tells the owner when and how to give the medicine to the animal at home. Sometimes, though, the drug must be given as an injection. The veterinarian gives these injections to the animal in the treatment room.

The veterinarian uses antibiotics in cases of virus disease, too. The drug does not control the virus, but it does prevent other infections from developing.

The veterinarian has a whole shelf of medicines to get rid of parasites on the outside of the animal's body. There are powders, sprays, soaps, shampoos, and liquids to get rid of fleas, lice, mites, and ticks. Each one works in a different way and is best against one type of parasite. The veterinarian chooses the one that he feels will do the job best and is safest to use.

The animal doctor handles an animal that is infected with parasites very carefully. The parasites spread easily from one animal to another. He must be sure that the parasites he removes from one animal do not get on to the fur or skin of the next animal he treats.

There are also several drugs that the veterinarian uses to get rid of worms inside the body. Often he uses a combination of two drugs. One drug breaks the grip with which the worms are attached. The other drug flushes the worms out of the animal's body.

Many veterinarians suggest two de-worming treatments, a few weeks apart. In this way they can be sure that all the worms are gone.

Worms are spread from one animal to another by the eggs they lay. The eggs leave the body of the sick animals in their feces (bowel movements). When a healthy animal touches the feces, the egg gets into his fur. In time, the animal licks his fur clean and swallows the tiny egg. Once inside the body, the egg grows and changes until it becomes a full-sized worm.

The veterinarian explains to the owner of the diseased animal how worms spread and grow. He stresses the importance of keeping the animal clean. And he gives advice on how to avoid worms in the future.

Animal patients that have broken bones, cuts, or other problems require quite different treatments. The doctor sets and holds broken bones in place with splints or a cast. He has drugs that will help dogs that are vomiting and suffering with diarrhea. When the skin is badly cut or torn, the veterinarian uses a thin needle to stitch and hold the edges of the skin together. He applies medicinal

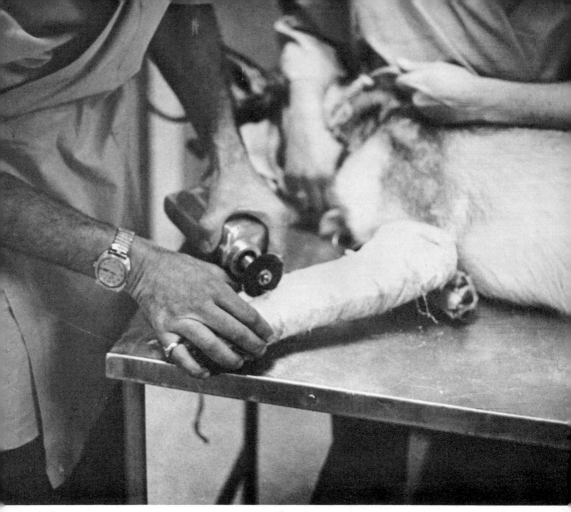

*The veterinarian uses a small power saw to cut the plaster cast
off the leg of a dog after the broken bone has mended.*

creams to wounds and skin sores. He cleans the ears and eyes of
sick pets with an array of drugs and instruments. The veterinarian
uses dental tools to clean the animal's teeth.

Modern veterinary science has given the doctor an amazing

Melvin Berger

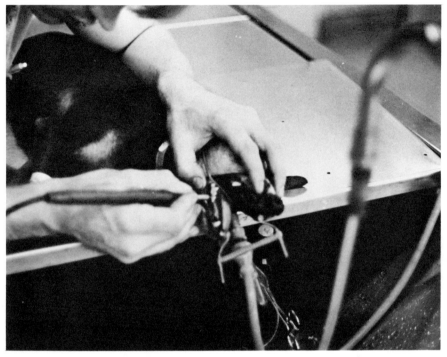

The veterinarian must also be part dentist.
Here he cleans a dog's teeth.

number of ways to prevent, control, and cure disease. And it is in
the treatment room of the animal hospital that he brings together
all that he has learned, and all of his skills, to provide the best
possible medical care for each pet.

THE HOSPITAL LABORATORY

The little puppy on the table in the examining room was a sad sight. She looked weak and wobbly. Her coat was dull and looked as though it had never been combed. Her eyes were red and watery. She was sneezing and coughing.

The veterinarian who examined her thought of several diseases that might cause these symptoms in the seriously ill dog. But the more he studied the animal, the more he was convinced that the dog was badly infected with worms.

It is a simple medical matter to get rid of worms. But before he could begin to treat the dog, he had to know exactly what kind of worms she had.

For this kind of information, the doctor needs the help of the scientists who work in the hospital laboratories. The modern veterinarian depends on the hospital laboratory to tell him more about an animal's condition than he can find out in the examining room. The laboratory scientists do all sorts of tests on samples of blood, urine, feces, and tissue that are taken from the sick animal by the veterinarian. These tests tell if the animal is sick, the extent of his illness, and the exact cause. Later, the laboratory scientist tells the veterinarian how well his treatment is working.

The doctor told the owner to return the next day with a sample of the dog's feces. Worms lay eggs which pass out of the dog's body in his feces. By examining the feces, the laboratory scientist can learn whether there are worms present. By studying the eggs under a microscope, he can tell what kind they are.

As soon as the owner brings in the sample, the veterinarian sends it to the laboratory. The scientist there places some of the sample in a test tube and adds some chemicals. The chemicals cause the food remains to sink to the bottom and any eggs that are present to float on the surface.

Then the scientist takes some of the surface liquid and places it on a glass slide. He examines it through his microscope. As he adjusts his microscope, he sees a number of eggs on the slide. Quickly he identifies the type of worms that lays eggs of this size and shape. He writes up his observations on a laboratory report form and sends it to the veterinarian. The veterinarian reads the report and begins treatment to get rid of the worms that are making the puppy sick.

During a day at work in an animal hospital, the veterinarian may take several small samples of blood from his animal patients.

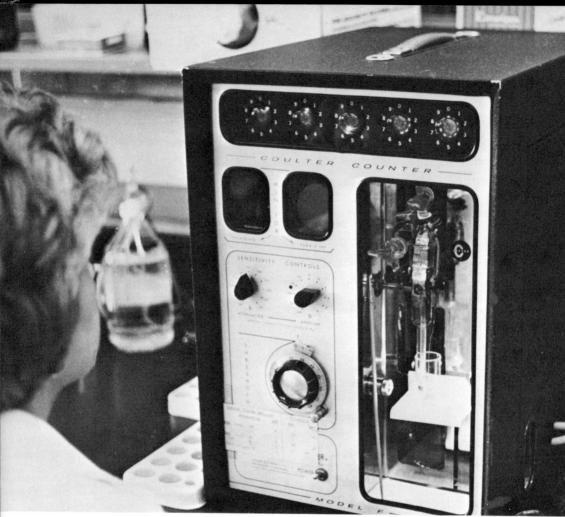

The worker in the hospital laboratory watches the automatic machine that counts the number of blood cells.

These may be from animals that are brought in for a visit or from animals that are staying in the hospital for treatment.

The veterinarian sends these blood samples to the laboratory. He writes down the tests that he wishes to have done on the blood.

The laboratory scientist performs the tests and sends back a report. The report not only tells the doctor if there is a disease of the blood, but it tells if there is a disease anywhere in the body that has led to changes in the blood.

There are over fifty different blood tests that can be done in the laboratory of an animal hospital. In one basic test, the scientist counts the number of cells in the blood. He places a measured sample of blood into an electronic counter. This special equipment automatically counts each of the individual cells.

The laboratory scientist studies a sample of blood through the microscope. She uses the counter at her left hand to record the numbers of the different types of cells.

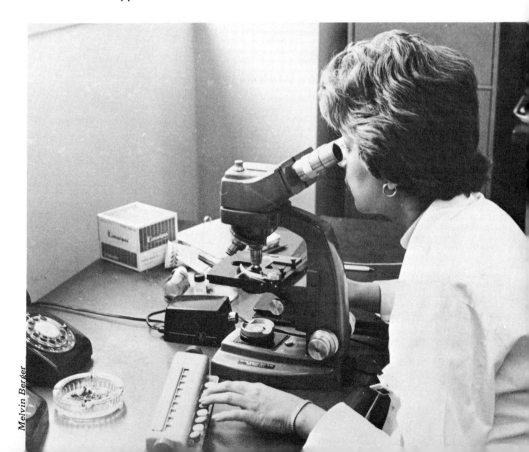

Melvin Berger

The veterinarian may want more than just a count of the cells. He may want to know the numbers of different kinds of blood cells that are present. The laboratory scientist then spreads a sample of blood on a glass slide, or makes a blood smear. He examines the slide under his powerful microscope. As he sees the different kinds of cells that are present, he presses buttons on a counter that records the number.

To study each part of the blood by itself, the scientist places a small blood sample in a thin tube. He puts the tube into a centrifuge, a machine that spins the sample around at great speeds. The heavier cells in the blood are forced down to the bottom of the tube. They are separated from the lighter, liquid part of the blood.

Most of the other blood tests find the amount of different substances that are in the blood. Usually, the laboratory scientist adds chemicals to the sample. As the chemicals react with the substances in the blood, the color of the sample changes. The color tells the scientist how much of each substance is present. Automatic machines measure the final color and tell the exact amount of the substance in the blood.

There are similar tests of urine samples to learn the number and types of cells that are present. These tests also show up any strange substances that may be in the urine of the animal.

The veterinarian turns to the laboratory when he wants to confirm a diagnosis of an animal's illness that he feels is due to bacteria. The laboratory scientist will be able to identify the particular bacteria that may be causing the illness.

The veterinarian rubs a cotton swab around the infected area. He sends the swab to the laboratory. The laboratory worker

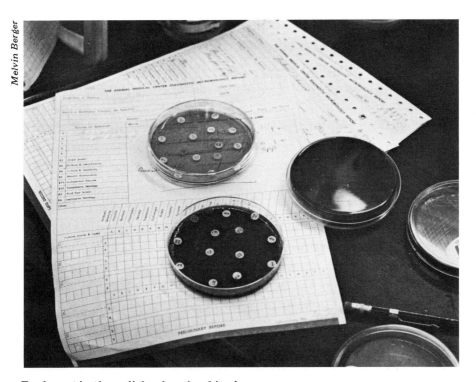

Melvin Berger

Each spot in these dishes is a tiny bit of
a different drug. Bacteria are grown in the dishes to see
which drugs will kill that type of bacteria.

smears the swab on a solid jelly, which is a food on which most
bacteria will live and grow. The jelly is in a round dish made of
clear plastic. He places a cover on top of the dish to prevent other
bacteria from falling onto the jelly.

As the bacteria grow in the dish, the scientist studies them under
his microscope. He checks their appearance and how they grow.

This information tells him the type of bacteria that are in the sample. He reports his findings to the veterinarian. The veterinarian decides on the treatment he will follow.

Sometimes the laboratory scientist is asked to find the drug that will work best against a certain type of bacteria. He smears the material that contains the bacteria on a jelly that has little spots of different drugs. In a few days, the bacteria cover most of the dish. But around one or more drugs there are clear spots. These drugs prevent the growth of the bacteria. The laboratory report lists the drugs that would be helpful in treating the animal.

One part of the hospital laboratory is devoted to pathology, the science of the nature and cause of disease. The scientists that work here are called pathologists. They work very closely with the veterinarians that operate on animals in the surgery unit of the hospital.

During some operations, the surgeon must know if the tissue is healthy or diseased, normal or cancerous. In a few cases he must know before he can proceed with the operation. While the animal is on the operating table, he takes a little snip of tissue. He sends it to the pathologist in the laboratory and waits for the report to come back.

The pathologist works with great speed. The sample of tissue from the surgeon is too thick to be examined under his microscope. He must make thin slices of the tissue. But the tissue is soft. It cannot be sliced. The quickest way to make it hard is to freeze it. Solid tissue is easy to slice.

The pathologist sprays the sample with a special chemical. In seconds it is frozen. The pathologist places the solid tissue in a cutting machine, called a microtome. It is similar to a salami slicer

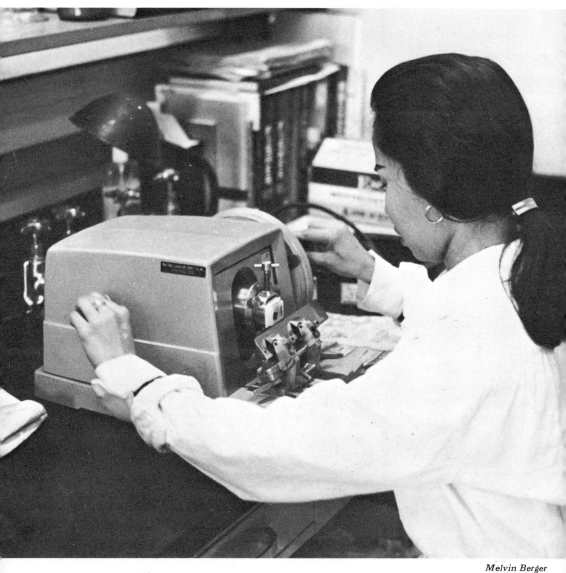

This machine is a microtome.
It is used to cut very thin slices of tissue
for study under a microscope.

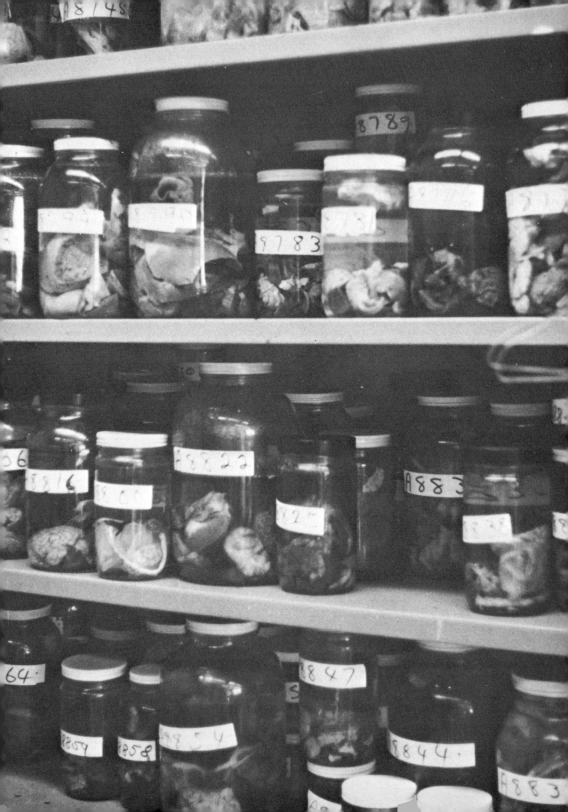

in a delicatessen. The machine cuts the tissue into very fine, thin slices.

The scientist places several slices on a glass slide. He sets it in his microscope. He studies the sections of tissue, looking at the size and shape and color of the cells. Are any cells abnormal? In what way are they different from normal cells?

In about five minutes, the pathologist completes his study of the tissue. By telephone or by messenger, he sends his report to the surgeon. The report tells the condition of the tissue. On the basis of the report, the surgeon decides how to proceed with the operation.

Sometimes the tissue or organ that is removed from the animal during an operation is sent to the pathologist. The pathologist studies this material to learn all he can about disease. He looks for the changes brought about by disease. He sees the differences between healthy and diseased tissue. He searches for the effects of drugs and other treatments. He looks for clues that will help the veterinarian treat similar cases in the future.

In some cases, an animal does not recover from an accident or from disease. When such an animal dies at the hospital, the veterinarian may have to ask the pathologist to help him discover the exact cause of death. If the veterinarian is not sure why the animal died, he performs an autopsy. He looks into the dead body for signs of disease. Sometimes he can see the cause immediately. Other times he removes some parts or organs of the body and gives them to the pathologist. The pathologist has the special laboratory equipment and special training to be able to find out exactly what led to the animal's death.

The pathologist keeps diseased organs that
he has taken from dead animals
on the shelves of his laboratory.
He studies them to learn more about disease.

Melvin Berger

Most pathologists are veterinarians who have done advanced work in this branch of veterinary medicine. Some of the other laboratory scientists are also veterinarians. Others are just highly trained laboratory technicians. In any case, they are all vital to the work of an animal hospital.

THE X-RAY ROOM

A girl carried a cat wrapped in a blanket into the waiting room of the hospital. The animal had just been hit by a car. The girl was very frightened and worried.

Without wasting a moment, the receptionist picked up a small microphone on her desk and said, "Doctor, could you come to the waiting room, please. Emergency." The announcement could be heard all over the hospital.

The veterinarian stopped what he was doing. He rushed to the waiting room and took the frightened girl and her pet to an examination room.

The cat was lying very still. It was hard to tell how badly it had been injured. The veterinarian immediately started his examination. He took the cat's temperature. He checked its gums. Pale gums would indicate that the cat was bleeding somewhere inside its body. Everything seemed to be all right.

While examining the cat, though, the veterinarian noticed that the left hind leg was bent in an unnatural way. He suspected a broken, or fractured, bone in the leg.

The veterinarian called for a set of X-rays of the leg. He wanted to see the X-rays so he could know for sure whether a bone was really broken. If he did find a fracture, he would use the X-ray pictures to decide how to set the bone so that it would heal and return to normal.

The doctor also asked for X-rays of the rest of the cat's body. They would tell him if there were any injuries to internal organs.

X-rays are invisible beams that are able to pass through many types of solid objects, including human and animal bodies. To get an X-ray picture, the veterinarian places a photographic plate behind the animal and sends X-rays through his body. The photographic plate is tightly wrapped in dark paper so that no light can strike it. But the X-rays pass through the paper wrapping and strike the plate.

When the plate is developed, it looks like the negative of a regular photograph. The thin parts of the body show up as dark areas, because they let all of the X-rays through to strike the plate. The bones and heavier parts of the body show up lighter in color, because they stop some of the X-rays and do not let them get to the plate. The result, then, is a shadow picture of the flesh and bones inside the body of the animal.

One of the hospital's workers helps the veterinarian take X-ray

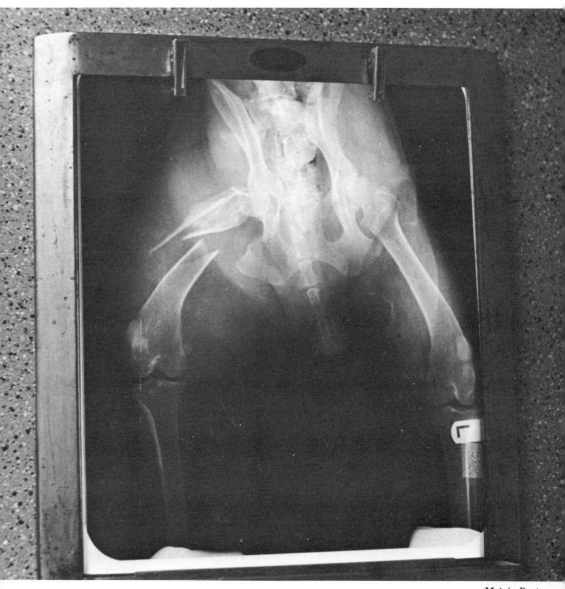

Melvin Berger

An X-ray picture of the badly smashed leg of a dog.

pictures of the cat. He wears a heavy apron that covers the entire front of his body and a pair of thick, heavy gloves. The apron and gloves are made with lead, which is one of the best shields against X-rays. Too much exposure to X-rays can injure or kill body cells. Therefore people who work with X-rays are always careful to protect themselves.

Everyone who works in the X-ray room wears a lead apron and gloves to protect him against the dangerous X-rays.

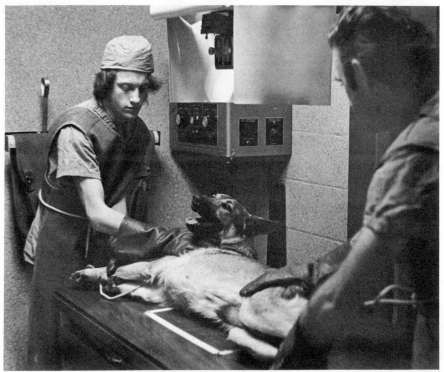

Melvin Berger

The veterinarian picks up the cat and with his assistant they head down the hall to a closed door. On the door is a big, bright red sign X-RAY ROOM. DANGER. DO NOT ENTER. This sign warns people to stay away from the dangerous X-rays.

The room is not in use right now and the men enter. It is dimly lit. Most of the space is taken up by a large, shiny black table in the middle of the room. The assistant places the cat on the table. Holding the cat in place with one hand, he moves an overhead metal box into position over the animal. The box is the actual X-ray machine. It will send the X-rays through the cat's body.

The assistant turns on a small light that is attached to the X-ray machine. He uses this light to focus the machine, and he moves it about until the light shines on the exact spot he wishes to aim the X-ray. The room is dimly lit so that this light can be clearly seen.

Then he takes a large photographic plate out of a box. It is wrapped in paper. He slips the plate into a slot in the table under the cat.

While the assistant holds the cat with his lead gloves, the veterinarian goes behind a protective metal screen. The controls of the X-ray machine are there. He presses a button. There is a soft whirr for a few seconds as the machine sends a stream of invisible rays through the cat's body, through the paper wrapping, and onto the photographic plate.

The veterinarian reenters the room. They rearrange the machine and move the cat. A fresh photographic plate is slipped beneath the animal. And again the veterinarian goes behind the metal screen and takes the X-ray picture. This is done as many times as is necessary to get all the pictures that the veterinarian needs. The assistant then takes the photographic plates into the dark room to develop them. The veterinarian puts the cat into an empty cage for a while.

Soon the X-ray pictures are ready. The assistant snaps them into a holder on the wall. He flicks a switch that lights the panel behind the X-ray pictures, bringing out all the details.

The veterinarian comes over to look at the X-rays. The bones of the cat's body show up as white lines. He sees a thin, dark line across a bone in the cat's left hind leg. His trained eye recognizes it as a fracture at once. He checks the other X-rays. No other problems.

The fracture is clean and straight, and therefore it is not too serious. The veterinarian places a plaster cast on the cat's leg. This will keep the bone in place so that it will be able to heal by itself.

The next day the girl comes to get her cat. She is delighted to learn that the cat will be all right. Over and over again she thanks the doctor for his help. The veterinarian is pleased too. He is always happy when he can relieve an animal's pain and bring comfort to its owner.

The veterinarian does not only look for broken bones or internal injuries with X-rays. He can also use X-rays as a tool to explore the cause of disease in animals. If he suspects that an animal has an enlarged heart, he can check with an X-ray. He looks for possible blockage in the intestines in the same way. He can pinpoint the exact size and location of internal growths, like cancers, with X-ray pictures.

One of the most valuable and frequently used tools in today's animal hospital is that amazing, invisible beam, the X-ray.

THE OPERATING ROOM

The veterinarian stands at the sink of the scrub room which is off to one side of the operating room. He rubs a powerful soap all over his hands and arms. He scrubs hard, as though he were trying to scrape away a layer of skin. He is about to perform an operation, and he must make sure that he will not bring any germs into the operating room.

After washing thoroughly, he takes a small, sterile brush from a sealed paper bag. He starts to scrub around his fingernails and knuckles. He rinses off the soap and starts again. More soap, more scrubbing, another rinse. Then, he dips his spotless hands into a deep basin that is filled with disinfectant.

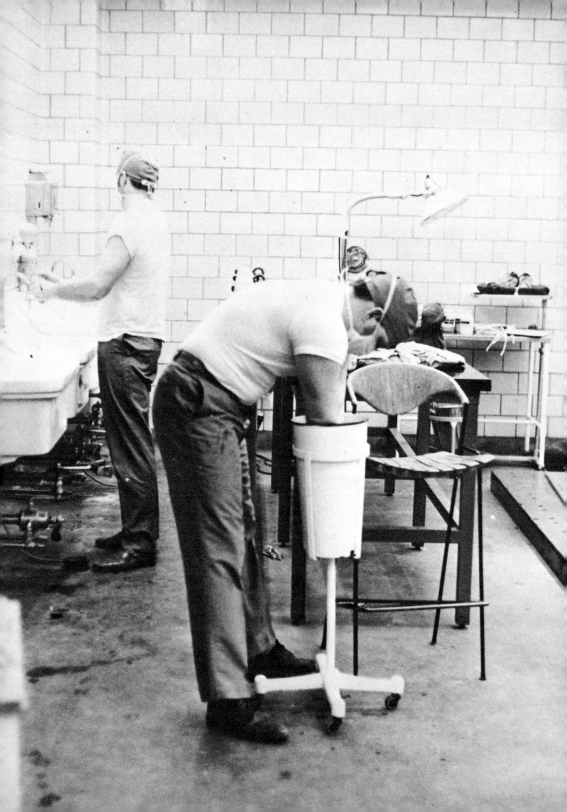

As he washes up, the veterinarian thinks about the operation that he will be performing in the operating room. Whether it is an operation to spay a female animal, to straighten out the bones in a fracture, to remove a diseased organ, to repair some internal injuries, or to search for the cause of a disease—the surgeon wants it to be safe and successful.

The careful scrubbing is one way to avoid infecting the animal with harmful bacteria. Another safeguard is for the surgeon to put on sterilized clothing for the operation.

The surgeon reaches for the bundle of clothes that is wrapped in heavy green cloth. The cloth is crushed and wrinkled. But it is far cleaner than the neat, ironed wash from a commercial laundry. The entire bundle of clothes has been scalded with hot steam under high pressure to kill any bacteria that might be on it.

The veterinarian unties the strings that hold the bundle together. He is careful not to touch anything else. Inside the package is a surgeon's gown, hat, and mask.

He picks up a corner of the folded cloth gown and straightens it out. Then, with an acrobatic wave of the hands, he tosses the gown into the air and slips his arms into the sleeves as it comes down around him. Twisting his body, he reaches for the strings and ties the gown closed in the back.

He puts on the hat and mask very carefully. They must not touch any surface in the scrub room that is not germ-free. From a sealed package, he takes out a pair of new rubber gloves. He pulls on these very thin, very tight gloves. They are another important safety measure to prevent infecting the animal during surgery.

While the veterinarian is scrubbing and dressing, an assistant

Two veterinarians prepare for surgery
in the scrub room. One is still washing,
while the other is already
dipping his hands and arms in disinfectant.

Melvin Berger

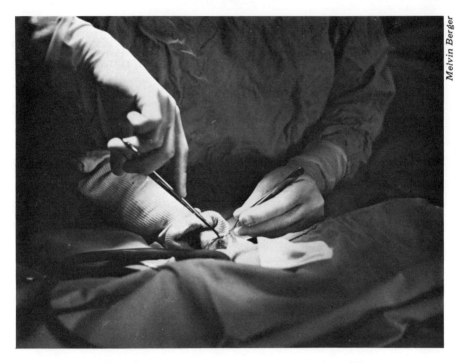

The powerful lights in the operating room shine on the place where the surgeon is working to repair a cat's fractured leg.

is getting the animal who needs surgery ready for the operation. The assistant gives the animal an injection that puts him into a light sleep. With an electric clipper he removes all the hair from the place where the surgeon will make the incision, or cut. He washes the whole area with a strong disinfectant.

Then the assistant brings the animal into the large, brightly lit operating room. He places the animal on the narrow, steel operating table in the center of the room. He straps the pet into the correct position for the surgery. The straps also hold the animal still during the operation.

The operating room has many cabinets that are filled with surgical equipment and drugs. The assistant checks the gas containers that are near the operating table. These gases, or anesthetics, are used to put the animal into a deep sleep for the operation.

The assistant also checks to see that the surgical instruments that the doctor will need during the operation are lined up correctly on the nearby metal table. He arranges the bright powerful overhead lights so that they shine right on the patient.

By now, the surgeon is ready too. He enters the operating room. He makes sure that everything is all set for the operation. The thin, rubber tube that is attached to the container of gas is placed into the animal's mouth. With each breath he takes, the pet breathes in the anesthetic. In minutes, the animal is in a deep sleep. He will not feel any pain or discomfort during the operation.

The surgeon now opens another package of wrinkled cloth. He takes out rectangles of material, called surgical towels, and spreads them over the body of the animal. He folds back the towels to expose the shaved area. Little clamps are placed on the towels to hold them in place. The only place left uncovered is where he will make the incision.

The veterinarian lifts off the cloth that covers the surgical tools that have been laid out for him. These tools are sterile. They will be sterilized again after the operation.

Everything is ready at last. The veterinarian picks up a tool that has a very short, sharp blade at one end. This is the scalpel, the surgeon's knife. Moving carefully but rather quickly, the surgeon makes the first cut into the animal's skin.

Back and forth the knife flashes under the bright lights. From time to time, the surgeon dabs at the oozing blood with a gauze pad. He cuts away layers of skin and tissue until he sees the bone or organ that he is after.

The most frequent operation that the veterinarian performs is to spay a female dog or cat. The veterinarian calls this operation a hysterectomy. In the operation the surgeon removes the animal's reproductive organs. It makes it impossible for her to become pregnant.

Owners who bring in their pet for a hysterectomy usually want to avoid the risk of unwanted litters of puppies or kittens. They may also want to protect the health of an animal that might not survive a pregnancy and birth, or they ask for the operation because a spayed animal tends to wander away from home less often. The similar operation performed on male dogs and cats is called a castration.

A simple hysterectomy or castration can be completed in about half an hour. The animal is usually kept in the hospital for a day or two, to be sure that no complications develop.

Another frequent operation is to repair a fracture. The veterinarian cuts through the flesh to the bone that is broken. He is guided to the exact spot by the X-rays that he took. He cleans away any infected tissue and any chips of bone. He brings together the two ends of the bone. Finally he places a plaster cast on the animal to make sure that the bones heal in the right position.

Modern veterinary surgeons have developed new methods of

The cat who is having a hysterectomy is almost completely covered with surgical towels. The pipe that leads to the animal's mouth is for the anesthetic.

Melvin Berger

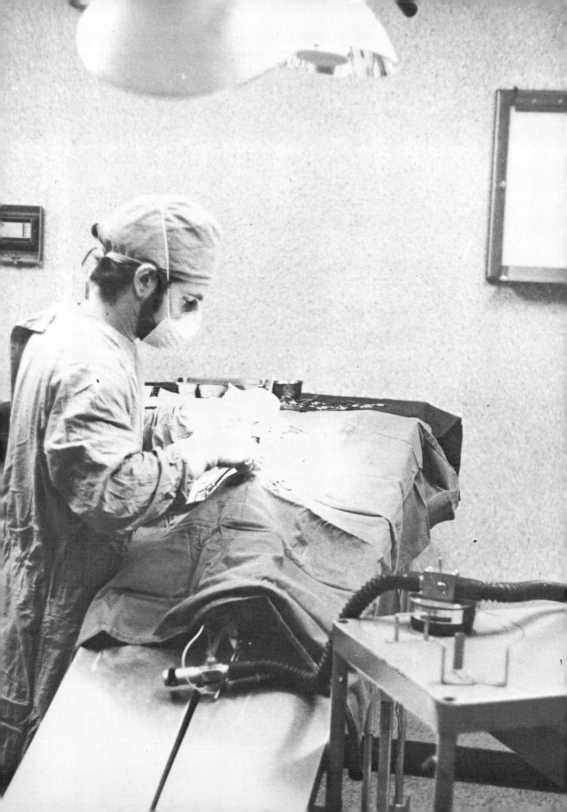

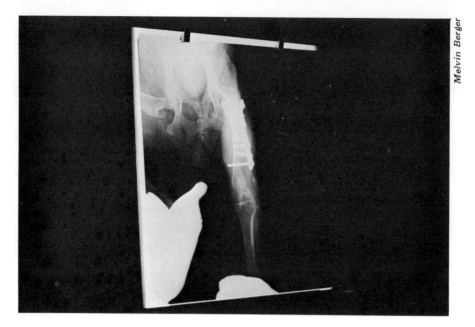

This X-ray picture shows the screws and plate that the surgeon placed in a dog's leg to repair a very bad fracture.

fixing bones that have been very badly smashed in accidents. They use metal screws and plates to restore the broken bones, so that the animal can walk normally again.

More complicated operations sometimes take several hours. If the surgeon suspects that something is blocking the intestines of the animal, for example, he must sometimes search for a long while before he finds the site of the trouble. If he needs to remove a diseased organ, he must work very carefully to repair all the damage that he makes by cutting it out.

He may have to interrupt the operation to get a report from the pathologist on tissue that he suspects may be diseased. In removing a growth, such as a cancer, he has to be certain that he removes all of the growth, yet cuts away as little healthy tissue as possible. It is also sometimes necessary to rebuild blood vessels, muscles, or nerves so that an animal can live despite a disease or injury.

Simple or complicated, the period of an operation is always a tense time. Surgery makes many demands on the skill and knowledge of the veterinarian. It is usually with a feeling of relief that the doctor goes into the final steps of the operation.

Once he is sure that everything inside the body of the animal is back in place, the doctor starts to pull together the outer layers of skin. He uses a small, sharp curved needle and surgical thread to sew together the skin along the incision. The series of separate stitches holds the skin firmly in place so that it will heal quickly.

The operation is over as soon as the last stitch is made. The doctor takes the tube from the animal's mouth, and the animal stops getting gas. The assistant gently carries the pet from the operating table to a nearby recovery cage.

In just a few minutes, the animal wakes up. At first he is shaky and wobbly. But before long, he is up and about. The veterinarian and other workers in the hospital keep a close eye on him, to make sure that he suffers no ill effects from the surgery.

If everything seems to go along as expected, the animal is brought back to his cage in one of the wards of the hospital. He continues to recover there.

If the operation was a simple one, like a hysterectomy, the pet may be permitted to go home in two days. After a more serious operation, such as bone surgery, the animal may be kept in the animal hospital up to two weeks.

The incision in the skin is healed completely about ten days after the operation. The veterinarian uses scissors to snip out the short

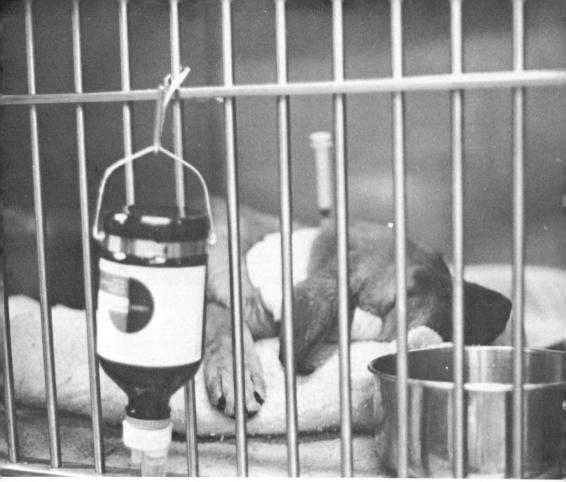

Melvin Berger

*It takes a little while for a dog to recover
after a serious operation. The veterinarian keeps a close watch
on him to make sure that he is all right.*

lengths of thread from the stitches. In a little while, the fur grows
back and it is hard to find the place where the cut had been made.
So great is the skill of today's veterinarians, that almost all patients recover quickly from surgery.

ANIMAL HANDLERS

Every animal hospital, large or small, has some special people who work there to assist the veterinarians. These workers are called animal handlers, animal aides or veterinary assistants. They help the veterinarians and the sick animals, the way nurses help doctors and human patients in ordinary hospitals.

People of all ages, from high school students to retired men and women, work as animal handlers. Many of the young handlers hope to become veterinarians when they grow up. They realize that working with a veterinarian and learning about the activities in an animal hospital will help them in their later career.

To qualify as an animal handler, you must be interested in animals and not be afraid of them. At the same time, you must not let your love for the animals get in the way of your work. A "gushy" attitude can lead to sloppy work. This can be bad for the animal and dangerous for the handler.

One of the main jobs of the animal handler is to restrain the animal. This includes holding him still during examination and treatment, taking him from one room to another, preventing his escape, and making sure that the animal does not injure himself, any people, or any other animals.

Old timers say, "No one is ever bitten during his first week as a handler." That is because a beginner is careful in his approach to animals that he does not know. But it is just as true to say that most handlers get bitten, scratched, or kicked at least once. Experienced animal handlers sometimes get careless and take risks that result in an injury of some sort.

Most handlers agree that a cat is more dangerous to handle than a dog. If a dog is muzzled, he is harmless. But a cat can scratch, as well as bite. Also, a cat's bite is a puncture and is more likely to become infected than a dog's bite, which is more of a tear in the skin.

Most handlers pick up a cat by grasping a handful of skin at the back of the animal's neck. When held this way, the cat can neither scratch nor bite. Most cats, in fact, curl up like tiny kittens when held in this grip.

The handler either carries a dog or leads it by a loop of rope around the animal's neck. If the dog seems dangerous, he may tie a muzzle made out of a long strip of gauze bandage over the dog's nose and mouth.

A particularly dangerous time for the handler is right after he

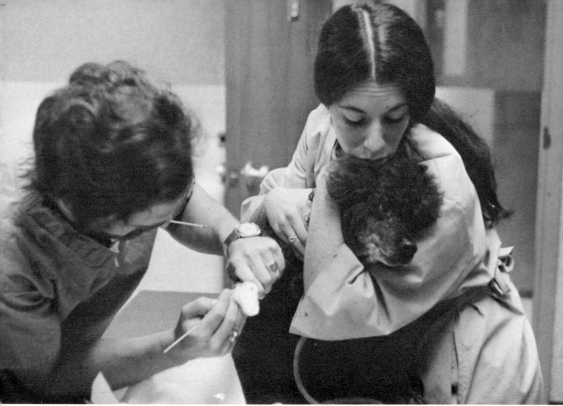

The handler holds the dog very tightly when she knows that the treatment may be hurting him.

has held an animal for a painful treatment by the veterinarian. The handler sees that the treatment is over and he relaxes. But the animal may still be in pain. It may attack either the handler or the veterinarian. The handler must always be ready for the unexpected.

Although the handlers know how to restrain all types of dogs and other animals, there are some animals that they do not like to touch. When a trained attack dog is brought to the hospital, for example, the handler and the veterinarian insist that the owner himself restrain the dangerous animal. In fact, the veterinarian will ask the owner of any animal that seems vicious or nasty to give that animal a sedative. A sedative makes the animal quiet and easy to handle.

The handlers also take care of the wards of the hospital. The wards are the rooms lined with cages for the animals that must stay in the hospital. An average ward may have twenty or thirty stainless steel cages of different sizes to hold the different types of animals. In each cage there is either a paper pad or a cloth blanket to make the animal more comfortable and to make it easy to clean the cage.

The veterinarian is ready to treat the black cat, and the handler gets her from the cage.

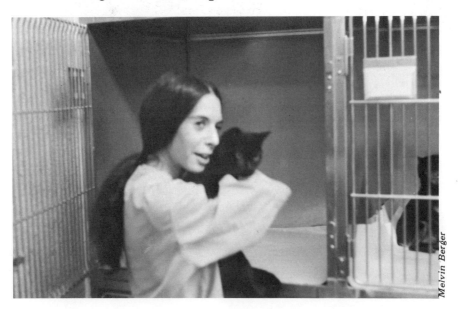

The handler makes sure that the wards and cages are as clean as possible. Some handlers begin their day by taking all of the animals out of their cages. They move them into the large exercise cages that are found in most wards.

Then he uses a high-pressure water hose to wash down the floors and walls of the ward. He scrubs the cages, inside and out. At the end of about two hours, the ward is spotless, and he returns the animals to their cages. During the day he keeps checking the cages and cleans up any mess that he sees.

Very often the handler is instructed by the veterinarian to give the animals their drugs. He walks around the ward with a cart of medicines. To give a liquid medicine, he usually holds the pet's head up and inserts a finger into his cheek, pulling out the lower lip. This forms a pocket, even though the animal's teeth are clamped shut. He pours or spoons the medicine into this pocket. It runs down between the animal's teeth, and he naturally swallows it.

To give an animal a pill, the handler actually holds its mouth open. He drops the pill as far back in the mouth as he can. Then, he pushes the pill down with his finger, forcing the animal to swallow it. Sometimes, the handler will mix the pill in with the food so the animal gets the medicine as he eats.

Some drugs can be given only by injection with a hypodermic needle. The veterinarian always gives the handler exact instructions on how to give each type of shot.

The handler also comes through the ward once a day with food for the animals. The usual food is a mixture of canned meat and dry meal. He opens cans of special foods for those animals that have been placed on diets of one kind or another by the veterinar-

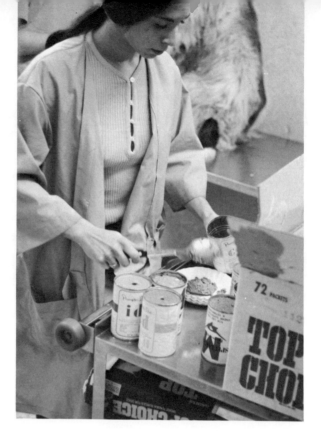

Chow time! The handler dishes out the food for all the animals in the ward. Some of the animals are given special foods.

ian. But most animals that are sick, or away from their homes, eat very little, if they eat at all.

Some large animal hospitals have a ward for the animals who have just had surgery or who are very seriously sick. One or two handlers with special training are on duty in this ward twenty-four hours a day. They keep constant watch over their patients. They look for a sudden change in the condition of the pets. They know how to handle most of the emergencies that might arise. The handlers here also know when they cannot meet a problem and it is necessary to call the veterinarian.

The list of the jobs that the handler does goes on and on. They prepare the animals for surgery. Oftentimes they assist during the operation. They clean and groom the animals in the hospital. They observe the animals and report on their condition to the veterinarians.

But the animal handler does more than help with the medical work of the hospital. He comforts the kitten that is terrified of being separated from its owner. He walks the dog who is stiff after surgery. He spends a few minutes amusing the puppy who is crying in its cage.

The handler, who combines medical work with warmth and kindness toward animals, is a most valuable member of the animal hospital team.

RESEARCH IN ANIMAL MEDICINE

Veterinary medicine is a growing science. Every year new discoveries advance the amount of knowledge and understanding that doctors have about animal diseases. The animal hospitals are always bringing in new methods of diagnosis and treatment, new drugs, and new medical tools.

Most of these new ways in veterinary medicine come from the research work of veterinary doctors. Each veterinarian at work in an animal hospital is also a research scientist. He is always adding to his knowledge by studying, observing, listening to others, and experimenting in his day-to-day work of treating sick animals.

Some animal hospitals follow special research projects. A group

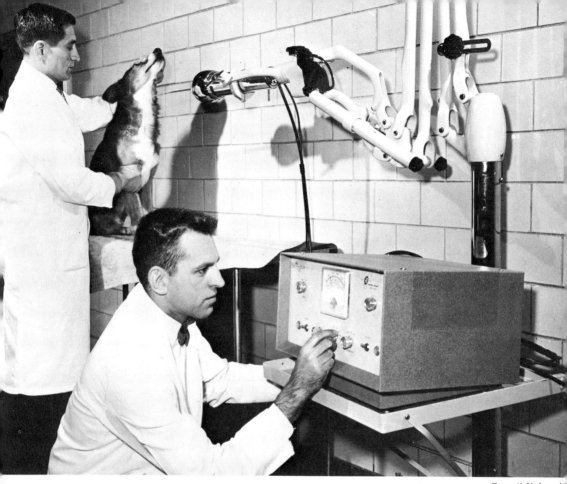

Cornell Universit

The veterinarians are using this advanced equipment in their research on the thyroid gland.

of veterinarians at work in a hospital may want to learn more about some aspect of veterinary medicine. A drug company may ask hospital veterinarians to test their new drugs and medicines. Some manufacturers of medical instruments and supplies want veterinarians to try out their new equipment. Any of these ideas can lead to research work in an animal hospital.

There are some veterinarians, though, that spend *all* of their time doing research in animal medicine. These doctors work in laboratories that may be part of an animal hospital or part of a veterinary college. They may be part of a drug manufacturing plant or a pet food factory. The veterinarians in these laboratories are mostly concerned with learning more about the causes, prevention, and cures of animal diseases.

The New York State Veterinary College of Cornell University in Ithaca, New York, is a center for veterinary research. Both teachers and students at the college work on many different research projects. In 1950 the college set up the Research Laboratory for Diseases of Dogs. It was the first laboratory devoted just to the study of dog diseases.

At that time many of the diseases of dogs were not understood very well. There were no good methods of recognizing the particular viruses or bacteria that were causing the diseases. And there were very few vaccines or drugs that the veterinarian could use to prevent or cure the diseases.

The major accomplishment of the early years of this laboratory was the development of a single vaccine that would prevent two widespread, serious diseases of dogs—distemper and hepatitis. In the past, about half of all the dogs that were brought to the veterinarian for treatment suffered from distemper. Today, largely due to distemper vaccine, the disease is under better control.

Laboratory scientists at the college have also developed a vaccine for leptospirosis, a disease that is often fatal to dogs. This highly contagious disease used to infect about one out of every four dogs.

The researchers have done even more than produce these new

vaccines. They have set standards to be used in testing all vaccines. They discovered the best time to give the dogs the vaccine. Their studies of newborn puppies have led to the invention of a puppy incubator. And they found a way to raise puppies who become separated from their mothers at birth.

They have made so many discoveries, in fact, that the scientists at the laboratory claim that almost every animal vaccine either originated at the laboratory or was discovered by someone who had once worked at the laboratory!

These scientists are now trying to develop new vaccines that will

Although this monkey will never wear glasses, the scientists are studying its eyes and vision.

Cornell University

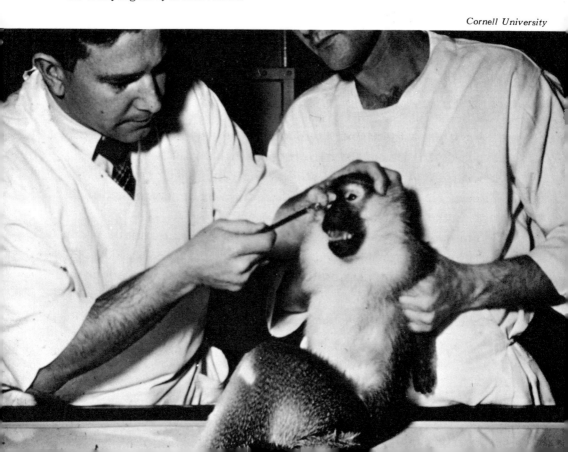

protect dogs against other types of viruses. They are most interested in the viruses that lead to kennel cough, to the deaths of newborn puppies, and to a type of chronic kidney disease that is found in older dogs.

The scientists who work with viruses have many difficulties and problems in their research. Viruses are so tiny that they cannot be seen through the ordinary laboratory microscopes. To see viruses, the scientist must use an electron microscope. This immense electronic instrument can make objects appear 200,000 times larger than they really are.

Viruses grow only in living cells. Therefore, the scientists have to find ways to grow the viruses in the laboratory, so they will have viruses to use for research. In the Diseases of Dogs Laboratory, the viruses are either grown in test tubes that have living cells or they are injected into eggs.

After the viruses grow in the test tube or in the eggs, the scientist has to separate the viruses from the other cells. He may spin the mixture of cells and viruses at great speeds in a machine called a centrifuge. As it spins, the heavier cell material goes to the bottom and the lighter viruses rise to the top.

Very often, the scientist will study a healthy dog that had been exposed to a virus in order to observe the disease it produces under laboratory conditions. He studies the general symptoms of the disease. He also tries to follow the viruses as they grow and multiply in the dog's body.

This work leads to studies with making a vaccine that will protect the dog against virus disease. The scientist has to study and choose from many possibilities. Should the vaccine be made from

A scientist examines viruses
through a giant electron microscope which
can magnify objects 200,000 times.

Cornell University

100

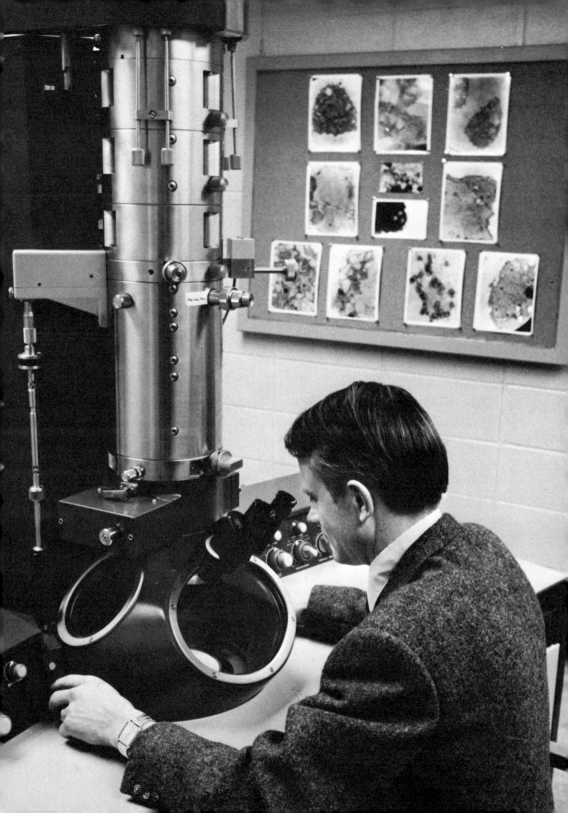

dead viruses or weakened viruses? If he uses weakened viruses, is there any danger that the viruses will infect the dog? How much vaccine should be given in each injection? At what age should the vaccines be given? How long will the protection last? Will the vaccine work in all dogs?

Many, many studies must be made before a new vaccine is developed to fight diseases in dogs.

One of the most valuable research tools at the laboratory is a group of pure-bred beagles that are completely free of disease and of disease-causing germs. Beagles were chosen because they are a small, short-haired, sturdy, and happy breed of dogs.

The dogs live in a separate kennel, away from the main building. A high, wire fence surrounds the kennel. There is only one gate and all supplies are unloaded and sterilized before they are brought into the building.

The laboratory staff are the only ones who are allowed to enter the kennel. The staff member must undress, shower, and put on special sterilized coveralls, boots, cap, and rubber gloves, before he can come into contact with the dogs. These garments are kept inside the building and are sterilized after each use.

The fact that the dogs are free of all disease-causing germs is very important to the researchers at the laboratory. When they use one of these dogs in an experiment, they can be sure that the only germs in the dog's body are those that they introduced. Much of the research at the laboratory could not be done without this world-famous colony of germ-free beagles.

Although most of the fifty scientists and workers on the laboratory staff study viruses and virus-caused diseases, there are other projects under way, as well. Some scientists at work want to learn more about several of the bacterial diseases. Some are studying the need for calcium and vitamin C in a dog's diet. And others are trying to increase the basic understanding of eye diseases, those that are inherited and those that are caused by infection.

From leading research centers, such as the Diseases of Dogs Laboratory, have come a long series of discoveries that have raised the health level of all animals. They have given the animal hospitals the knowledge and the drugs that they need to fight animal disease and sickness.

The veterinarian inspects baby chicks used to check the safety of some vaccines.

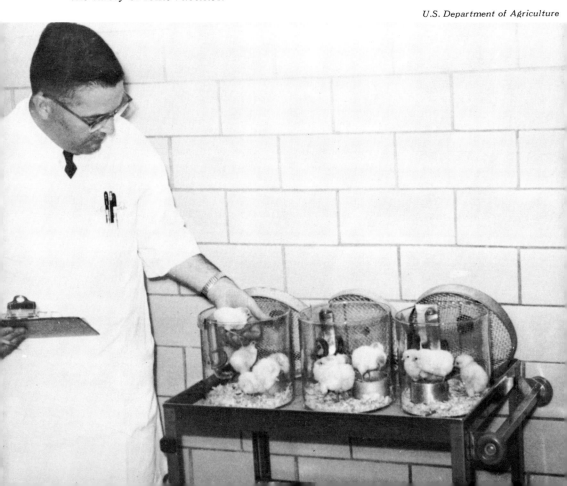

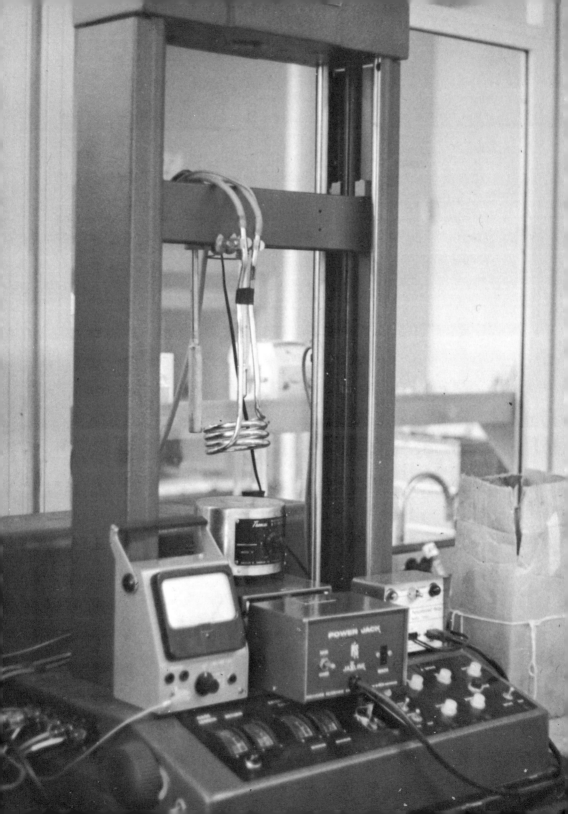

ANIMALS IN MEDICAL RESEARCH

There are a number of laboratories in which the scientists work to learn more about animal diseases. There are even more laboratories where scientists study animals and animal diseases in the hope that what they learn can be used to increase our knowledge of human disease.

One such laboratory is located in a large animal hospital in New York City. The main work of the scientists in this laboratory is to study the changes that take place in living beings as they age and grow old. They study factors that have to do with aging, from how much the skin can be stretched at different ages, to changes in the chemistry of the blood.

This machine is used to test how far skin can be stretched.
It has shown that young skin stretches more than old.

Melvin Berger

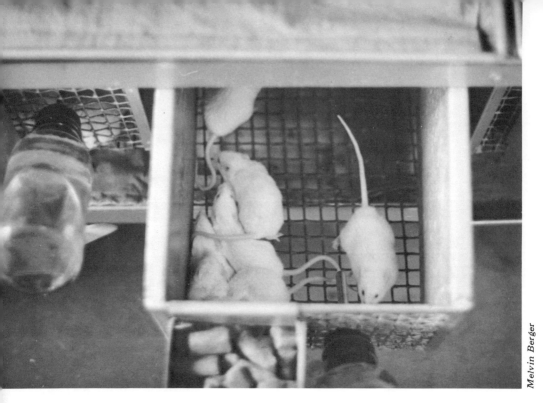

The mice are kept in drawerlike cages at the aging laboratory.

The research is performed on dogs, rats, mice, and fish. But the researchers are aware that discoveries they may make in their animal studies might some day lead to important breakthroughs in understanding aging in humans.

In one line of research, the scientists have been studying various types of fish. They want to learn why some fish live longer than others. The researchers are particularly interested in pinpointing the biological differences that are related to the life spans of the fish. They study the growth of fish and when they mature sexually, to see if there is any relationship to aging. They also study the body chemistry of aging fish.

The mouse is placed in a jar with a cloth soaked
in ether to put him to sleep.

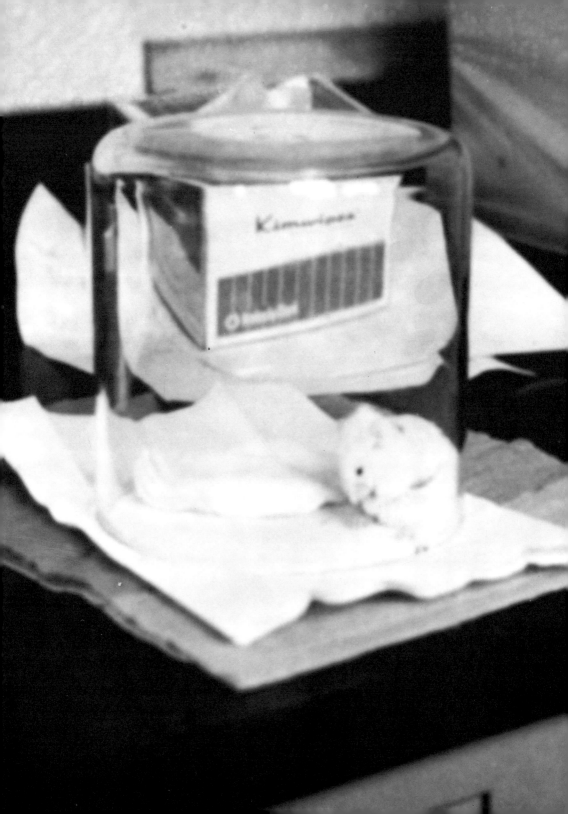

In another study, the researchers are trying to discover exactly how the blood changes as an animal ages. They carefully watch the growth of cells in blood serum taken from young and old animals.

If the researchers find differences in the blood serum their first job will be to identify the differences and separate the different factors. Then they will run experiments to learn more about the factors they have found. They will probably add the factors to a young animal's blood and observe the results. They will try to remove the factors from the blood of old animals and see if there are any changes.

Still another experiment being run at the aging laboratory compares the time it takes for a similar wound to heal in young and old animals. Researchers want to know what factors control the rate of wound healing.

The scientists have also collected samples of blood from dogs of various ages. They run tests of many kinds on these samples to see if they can find a chemical difference between young and old blood.

The experimenters in the aging laboratory have recently begun a research project to find the best way to transplant tissue from one animal to another. Transplants of tissue and organs have already been done in animals and humans with some success. They have helped to prolong the lives of those who received the transplants.

But there is always the fear that the body that receives the transplant will reject or destroy the foreign tissue. In human transplants doctors use large amounts of drugs to prevent the body from rejecting a heart or kidney transplant. Sometimes the trans-

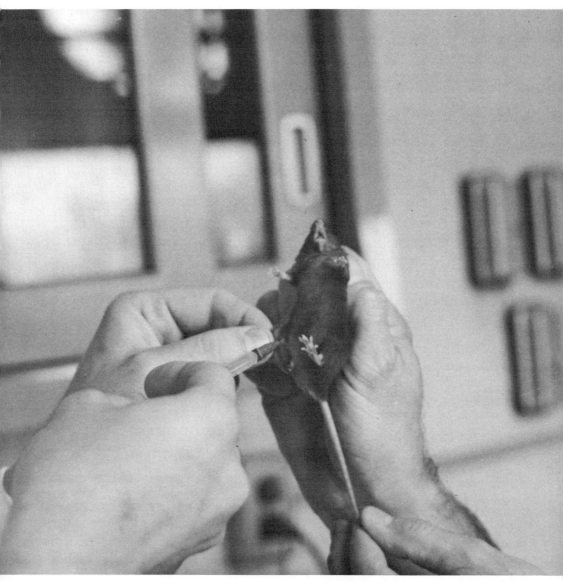

Melvin Berger

*The scientist injects a powerful anesthetic into the mouse
so that he will not feel any pain during the experiment.*

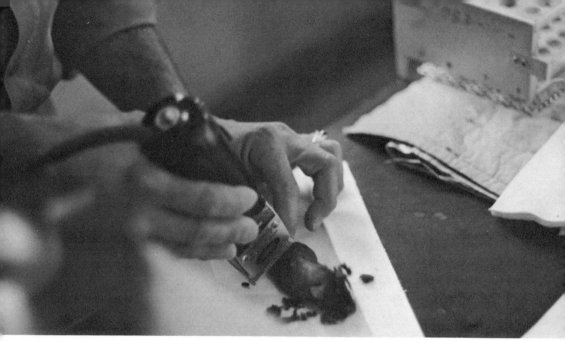

The scientist's helper uses an electric razor to shave off some of the fur on the mouse.

Using very sharp scissors, the researcher snips off about eight tiny bits of skin.

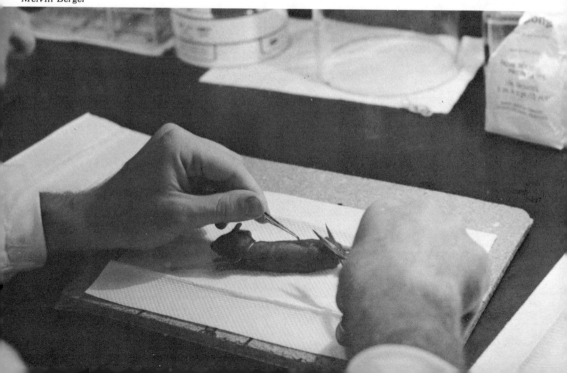

plant is accepted, but the patient becomes seriously sick or dies as a result of the powerful drug treatment.

The experimenters in the aging laboratory are trying to learn why some transplants work and some do not. And they want to be able to make successful transplants without the use of drugs.

The method they use is to transplant bits of skin from one mouse to another. To make it easier to see, they usually transplant skin from a white mouse onto a black mouse, and skin from a black mouse onto a white mouse.

The scientist uses a cloth that is soaked in ether to put a mouse to sleep. This is the donor mouse whose skin will be used for the transplants. He then injects a powerful anesthetic into the mouse. This is to make sure that the mouse will feel no pain during the experiment. An assistant shaves the animal's fur with an electric razor.

Placing the mouse on a paper towel, the scientist removes about eight tiny snips of skin. Since the donor mouse could not survive, it is quickly and painlessly sacrificed.

The scientist next takes the bits of skin and carefully cleans and trims them. He places each piece in a liquid solution in separate test tubes.

After a few days, several mice are prepared to receive the skin transplants. Each one is anesthetized, and an area of skin is surgically removed. The scientist takes the skin bits from the test tubes and bandages them into place. The mice are returned to their drawerlike cages.

About ten days later the scientist removes the bandages. By then he can tell whether the transplant is going to stay in place, or whether it will be rejected.

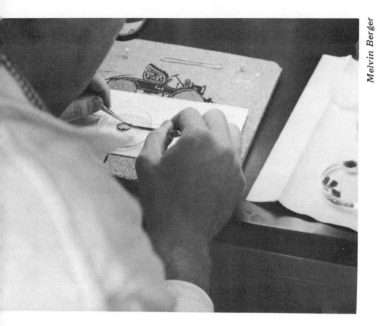

Each bit of skin is carefully cleaned and trimmed.

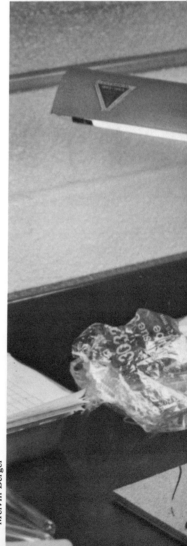

A laboratory assistant prepares the test tubes with the solution.
The bits of skin will be kept in these tubes.

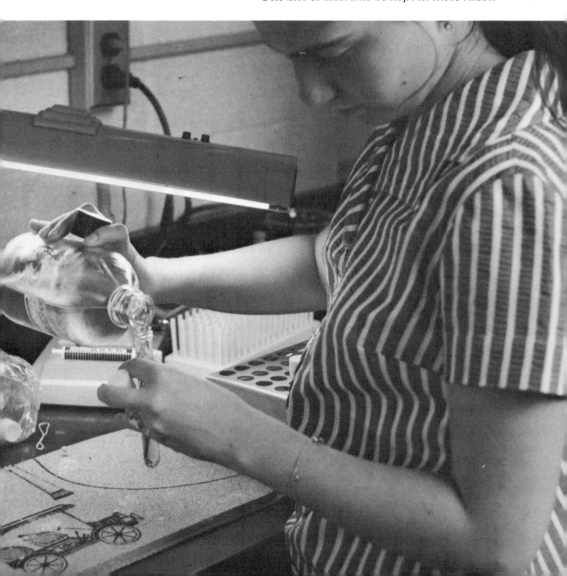

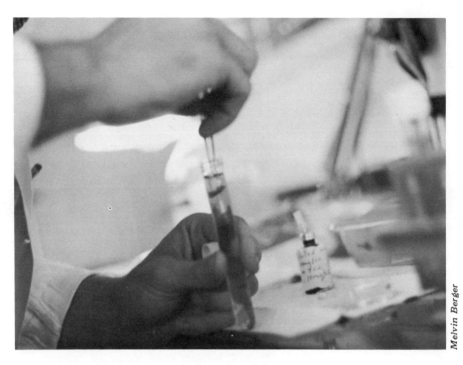

Each piece of skin goes into a separate test tube.

The scientist keeps a complete record in his notebook of the results of every experiment. Was the transplant a success? How long was it between when the skin was removed from one mouse and when it was placed on the other mouse? Which mouse was the donor, which mouse received the transplant? Was there any factor that might explain why this particular transplant was accepted or rejected?

It worked! The black patch on the mouse's body shows that the skin transplant is not being rejected.

Melvin Berger

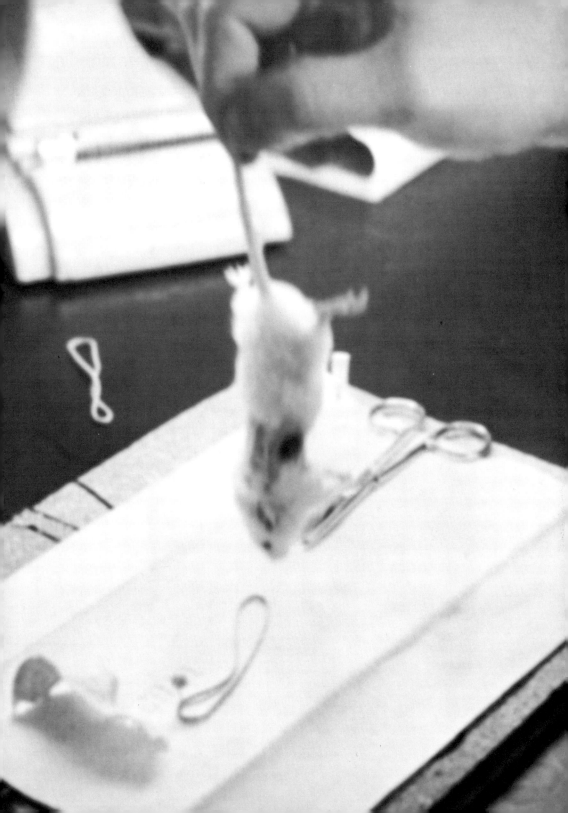

As this experiment goes on, the scientists are learning more about transplants. In time, perhaps, they will apply their methods to transplanting organs. And maybe, at some future date, someone will be able to use their findings to make possible the safe, sure transplant of human tissue and organs.

PRINCESS HAS PUPPIES

Princess is a very good-natured, playful, and loyal dog. Many people admire and praise her. From time to time, they have said to her owners, "If Princess ever has puppies, could we have one?"

Her owners decided to breed Princess. They waited until she was in her heat cycle and could become pregnant. Princess and a male dog, or sire, were brought together.

Bobby was the first to notice that Princess seemed to be getting fatter. She seemed less anxious to romp and play. Mother told Bobby that Princess probably would have a litter of puppies in a few weeks.

"Shall we take her to the animal hospital?" Bobby asked his mother.

"No. Princess can have her puppies without the help of the veterinarian. We will make a special box for her. She'll get used to

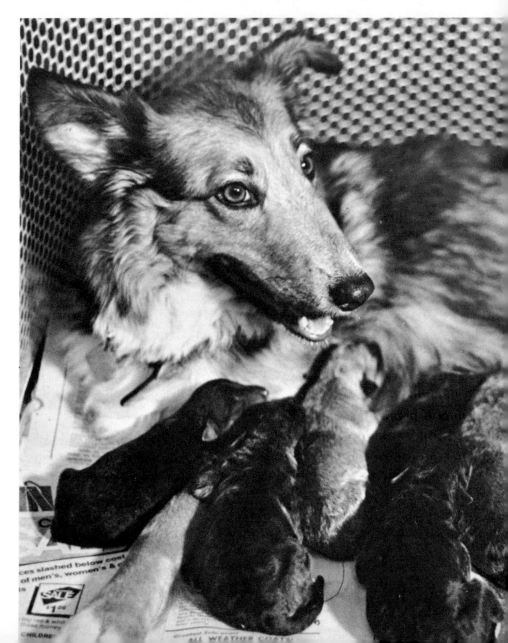

the box. When it's time for the puppies to be born, she will go there."

One day, while Bobby was in school, nine puppies arrived, one after the other. Princess started each puppy breathing by tearing

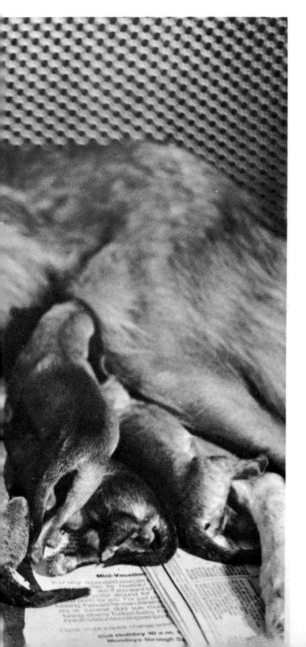

Princess has puppies!
The nine newborn pups snuggle
close to their mother.
Some are sleeping;
others are nursing.

Melvin Berger

ON THE FOLLOWING PAGES:
Bobby holds one of the puppies as
Princess licks it clean.

Melvin Berger

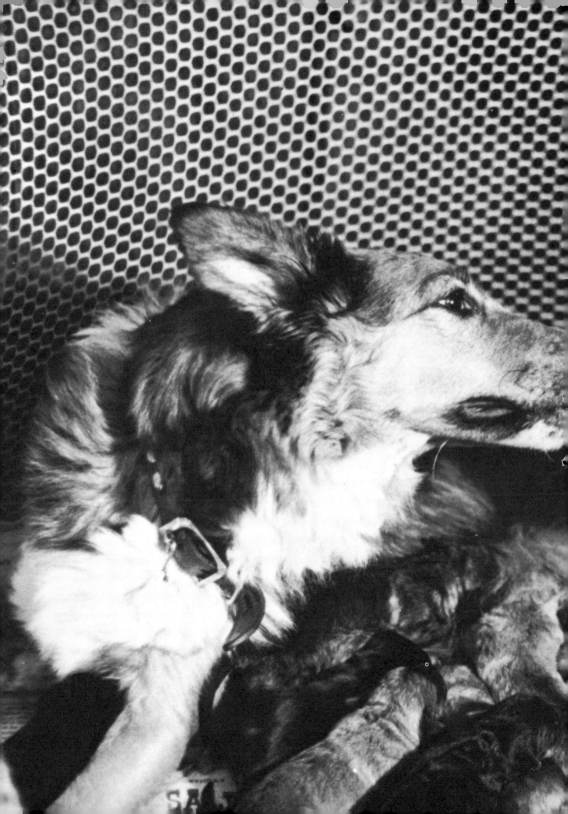

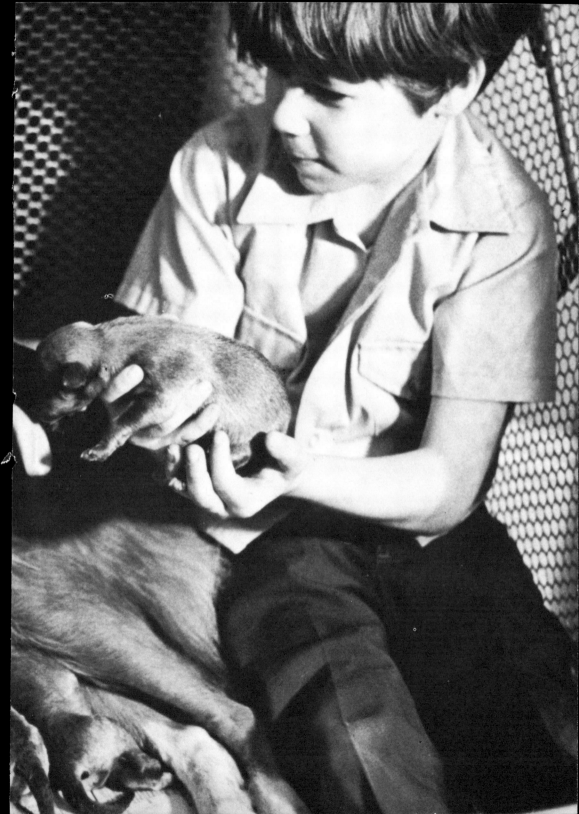

away the sac in which it was born. She licked each puppy clean from end to end.

Bobby was very excited. He wanted to let everyone know the good news. After he told all his friends about the puppies, his mother said that he could call the veterinarian.

The veterinarian was very happy to hear from Bobby. He told him that he should make sure that the puppies get plenty of milk from their mother. "It is important," he said, "that Princess get a good diet. And remember to bring the pups in for their first shots when they are about nine weeks old. Veterinarians don't want to see animals only when they are sick, you know. We want to help healthy animals grow well and stay healthy."

FURTHER READING

General books on veterinarians.

AMES, FELICIA, *The Bird You Care For.* New York, Signet, 1970

BRYANT, DORIS, *Pet Cats: Their Care and Handling.* New York, Ives Washburn, 1963.

DEAUTSCH, DR. H. J., and J. J. MCCOY, *The Dog Owner's Handbook.* New York, T. Y. Crowell, 1954.

WHITNEY, LEON F., *The Complete Book of Cat Care.* Garden City, Doubleday, 1953.

WHITNEY, LEON F., *The Complete Book of Dog Care.* Garden City, Doubleday, 1953.

Books on animal care.

MCCOY, J. J. *The World of the Veterinarian.* New York, Lothrop, Lee & Shepard, 1964.

MAY, CHARLES PAUL, *Veterinarians and Their Patients.* New York, Thomas Nelson, 1964.

INDEX

ABOUT THE AUTHOR

Melvin Berger was born in New York City. He was educated at City College; University of Rochester, where he received his Bachelor's Degree; Columbia University, where he earned his Master's Degree; and London University.

Mr. Berger loves to travel and it was during his travels that he made many side visits to laboratories. The idea for the series "Scientists at Work" grew out of these visits.

Mr. Berger lives with his wife and two daughters on Long Island, New York.

SCIENTISTS AT WORK